Diabetes: Caring for Patients in the Community

Edited by

Joan R. S. McDowell MN RGN SCM DN RNT

Lecturer, Department of Nursing and Midwifery Studies,
University of Glasgow, UK

Derek Gordon BSc MD FRCP

Consultant Physician in General Medicine, Diabetes and Endocrinology,
Law Hospital NHS Trust, Carluke, Lanarkshire, UK
Honorary Clinical sub-Dean, University of Glasgow, UK
Honorary Senior Lecturer, University of Edinburgh, UK

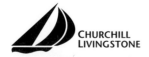
CHURCHILL
LIVINGSTONE

NEW YORK EDINBURGH LONDON MADRID MELBOURNE SAN FRANCISCO TOKYO 1996

CHURCHILL LIVINGSTONE
Medical Division of Pearson Professional Limited

Distributed in the United States of America by Churchill
Livingstone Inc., 650 Avenue of the Americas, New York,
N.Y. 10011, and by associated companies, branches and
representatives throughout the world.

First published 1996

ISBN 0 443 05295 6

British Library of Cataloguing in Publication Data
A catalogue record for this book is available from the British
Library.

Library of Congress Cataloging in Publication Data
A catalogue record for this book is available from the
Library of Congress

Note
Medical knowledge is constantly changing. As new
information becomes available, changes in treatment,
procedures, equipment and the use of drugs become
necessary. The editors/authors/contributors and the
publishers have, as far as it is possible, taken care to ensure
that the information given in this text is accurate and up to
date. However, readers are strongly advised to confirm that
the information, especially with regard to drug usage,
complies with latest legislation and standards of practice.

The
publisher's
policy is to use
paper manufactured
from sustainable forests

Produced by Longman Singapore Publishers (Pte) Ltd
Printed in Singapore

Diabetes: Caring for Patients in the Community

For Churchill Livingstone:

Commissioning editor: Ellen Green
Project manager: Valerie Burgess
Project development editor: Mairi McCubbin
Design direction: Judith Wright
Illustrator: Lee Smith
Project controller: Pat Miller
Copy-editor: Alison Bowers
Indexer: Tarrant Ranger Indexing Agency
Sales promotion executive: Hilary Brown

Contents

Contributors

Florence J. Brown RGN RMN RHV
Diabetes Nurse Specialist, Gartnavel General Hospital/Western
Infirmary, Glasgow, UK
  3. *Psychological care*

Derek Gordon BSc MD FRCP
Consultant Physician in General Medicine, Diabetes, and
Endocrinology, Law Hospital NHS Trust; Honorary Clinical Sub-
Dean, University of Glasgow; Honorary Senior Lecturer, University
of Edinburgh, UK
  4. *The patient with non-insulin-dependent diabetes mellitus*
  5. *The patient with insulin-dependent diabetes mellitus*
  8. *The patient with diabetic complications*
  12. *The organisation of diabetic care*

June Gordon BSc SRD
Senior dietitian, Aberdeen Royal Infirmary
Foresterhill, Aberdeen, UK
  6. *Dietary advice*

David M. Matthews BSc (Med Sci) MB ChB FRCP Edin FRCP Glas
Hairmyers and Stonehouse Hospitals NHS Trust,
Stonehouse Hospital, Lanarkshire, UK
  1. *What is diabetes?*

Joan R. S. McDowell MN RGN SCM DN RNT
Lecturer, Department of Nursing and Midwifery Studies,
University of Glasgow, UK
  2. *Diagnosis and screening for diabetes*
  5. *The patient with insulin-dependent diabetes mellitus*
  7. *Monitoring diabetes*

Christine M. Skinner BSc (Hons) DPODM MCLS SR CL
Lecturer, Division of Podiatry, Caledonian University,
Southbrae Campus, Jordanhill, Glasgow UK

Frank Sullivan PhD FRCP MRCGP
Senior Lecturer in General Practice, Glasgow University,
Woodside Health Centre, Barr Street, Glasgow, UK

Preface

Why write another book on caring for people with diabetes? We felt there was a need for a book that caters for the members of the primary health care team who in recent years have become more actively involved in the management of such people. While there are many books around on the subject, few have been specifically written for the care of the person with diabetes at home.

In addition, we both feel strongly that clinical practice should be based on a sound knowledge of principles. Within health care professionals there is the desire to produce 'knowledgeable, critical thinkers'. Such people do not follow blindly, but rather question current practice and seek to change this in the light of research. Hence each chapter has references for further pursuit of study.

The content of the book has arisen from teaching community nurses over several years. A successful course for Practice Nurses organised through the Department of Nursing and Midwifery Studies, University of Glasgow, has also been influential in determining content. Course evaluation has allowed us to determine the important topics and areas of knowledge that are most pertinent to the primary health care team.

We have attempted to make the text as readable as possible by incorporating case studies of real situations. We have developed principles of practice around these clinical case studies and have founded these upon research, where possible. Principles of good practice have been determined where there is as yet no current research available.

We have discussed the important findings of the Diabetes Control and Complications Trial (DCCT) research group and the UK Prospective Diabetes Study. The provision of diabetic care in the UK is influenced not only by improving clinical understanding of the disease but also by powerful political lobbies. We have therefore also described the important influences upon the provision of diabetes care that have resulted from the St Vincent Declaration.

We would like to thank our spouses and families for their support and encouragement through the many hours spent in front of the word processor. We acknowledge with gratitude the sterling work of the contributors who have devoted much time and effort to this enterprise. We have enjoyed working with them. We also wish to thank Julian Hodgson, Librarian and Janice Bryson, Postgraduate Secretary, Law Hospital NHS Trust for their time and effort in undertaking literature searches. Thanks must also go Eamon Shanley, Senior Lecturer in the Department of Nursing and Midwifery Studies, University of Glasgow and to Lesley Whyte, Lecturer in Community Health Studies, Glasgow Caledonian University for their support and advice.

We hope you enjoy reading this book, that it will influence your practice and that you will return to it many times in the future.

1996   J. McD.

D. G.

What is diabetes?

David Matthews

■ CONTENTS

WHAT IS DIABETES?

Definition

Diabetes mellitus is a chronic condition affecting between 1 and 2% of the general population. The management of patients with diabetes therefore poses a formidable challenge to the Primary Health Care Team. Diabetes mellitus comprises a group of diseases characterised by hyperglycaemia due to deficiency or diminished effectiveness of insulin. This results in a disorder of carbohydrate metabolism. Fat, protein and mineral metabolism can also be affected. Its importance as a disease is due to the irreversible tissue damage which results mainly from poor metabolic control.

Diabetic retinopathy is the commonest cause of blindness in persons aged under 60 years in the UK. One third of patients on programmes for the management of end-stage renal failure have diabetes. Having diabetes makes a person 2–3 times more likely to have a major vascular event such as myocardial infarction or stroke. Around 50% of patients having amputations for non-traumatic reasons have diabetes (Department of Health & British Diabetic Association 1995).

The resultant increased morbidity and mortality from diabetes is plain to see and explains why diabetes is a major consumer of health care resources world-wide.

Classification

There are various classifications of diabetes (Table 1.1). Non-insulin-dependent diabetes (NIDDM) or Type 2 is the commonest, representing around 80% of all diabetics. Insulin-dependent diabetes (IDDM) or Type 1 makes up most of the remaining 20%. Maturity onset diabetes of the young (MODY) and secondary diabetes are relatively uncommon and account for less than 1% of cases. However it is important to identify patients with secondary diabetes so that treatment can be directed to the underlying cause.

Diabetes in association with other genetic syndromes is also very rare. In these instances, diabetes is another burden which these people have to bear.

Table 1.1 Classification of diabetes

- Primary

Type 1 Insulin-dependent diabetes mellitus, IDDM
Type 2 Non-insulin-dependent diabetes mellitus, NIDDM
MODY, maturity onset diabetes of the young

- Secondary to other disorders

1. Pancreatic disease	chronic pancreatitis
	haemochromatosis
	pancreatectomy
	carcinoma of pancreas
	cystic fibrosis
2. Endocrine disease	acromegaly
	Cushing's syndrome
	phaeochromocytoma
	gestational
3. Drugs	thiazide diuretics
	corticosteroids

- Associated with genetic syndromes

Friedreich's ataxia
muscular dystrophies
Down's syndrome
Diabetes insipidus, diabetes mellitus, optic atrophy and deafness (DIDMOAD)

Insulin-dependent diabetes mellitus

The hallmark of IDDM is a dependence on exogenously injected insulin to prevent ketosis and maintain life. Without injected insulin, patients with IDDM die! This was the situation before the discovery of insulin in 1921. Some died very quickly over a matter of days. Others struggled along miserably for three or four years by eating almost starvation type diets (Bliss 1983). In IDDM, therefore, there is an absolute deficiency of insulin.

Case Study 1.1   *DKA case*

A 10-year-old boy is noticed to leave the classroom to go to the toilet more often than usual in the few days before taking seriously ill with a pyrexial illness and intermittent vomiting. His GP diagnoses urinary tract infection and prescribes antibiotics. Over the next 48 hours his condition deteriorates with continued vomiting and altered consciousness. When he proves unrousable his parents take him to the local casualty department where he is found to have diabetic ketoacidosis. He is admitted to the children's ward where, after intravenous fluids and insulin, he recovers. He will require insulin injections now for the rest of his life.

This case study is a fairly representative example of a newly diagnosed patient with IDDM presenting in diabetic ketoacidotic coma. Before the discovery of insulin such a presentation was lethal. Insulin saved this child and he will be dependent on self-injected insulin for the rest of his life. Withdrawal of insulin would rapidly cause further ketoacidosis, and he should be told never to stop his injections.

Non-insulin-dependent diabetes mellitus

This type of diabetes is the commonest form world-wide and there is no requirement for insulin to prevent ketosis and preserve life. The majority of patients can be managed by dietary means alone. Sometimes oral hypoglycaemic drugs are required in addition to diet. Most patients are over the age of 40 years when diagnosed. The main associated feature is obesity and in such people the body tissues are relatively resistant to the effects of insulin, thus causing elevation of blood glucose. By reducing body weight many patients can make carbohydrate tolerance almost normal.

There is a subgroup of patients however who are not obese and who have a relative deficiency of insulin. They cannot secrete enough insulin to cope with the carbohydrate load they consume. The pathological process in the islets of Langerhans in the pancreas is quite different from IDDM—they do not have autoimmune damage to the pancreas. However, these patients might eventually require insulin therapy although they will not be classified as having IDDM.

Maturity onset diabetes of the young (MODY)

This is a rare inherited form of diabetes which usually arises in teenage years and despite the young age at presentation, does not require insulin treatment. Most patients have a family history, with autosomal dominant inheritance. Recent molecular genetic research has shown several defects including a mutation in the glucokinase (GCK) gene located on the short arm of chromosome 7. These patients might be assumed to have IDDM because of their age at presentation. However they have a diabetes managed like NIDDM and are certainly not dependent on insulin (Tattersall 1991).

Secondary diabetes

This type of diabetes is secondary to other disease processes which cause either pancreatic damage or production of hormones which antagonise the action of insulin (Table 1.1).

Pancreatic disease

The pancreas can be damaged as a result of frequent bouts of pancreatitis often precipitated by alcohol abuse or the presence of gallstones in the common bile duct.

The inherited condition of haemochromatosis causes iron to be deposited in the pancreas and this in turn causes pancreatic damage and diabetes. This condition is associated with gradual pigmentation of the skin—hence the common clinical name 'bronze diabetes'.

The presence of carcinoma within the pancreas can also cause destruction of normal insulin-secreting cells resulting in the development of diabetes. Pancreatic disorders causing diabetes usually require treatment with insulin.

Case Study 1.2

A 73-year-old woman presents with a 9 kg (1.5 stone) weight loss associated with nausea, polydipsia, polyuria and vulvitis. 2% glycosuria is found and her random blood glucose is 19.7 mmol/l. Diabetes mellitus is diagnosed and she is treated with dietary measures as well as glipizide 2.5 mg to relieve her symptoms quickly. She returns three weeks later. Her glycosuria has disappeared, her blood glucose has fallen to 9.1 mmol/l but her weight has fallen by a further 2 kg.

It is unusual to be nauseated with primary diabetes, and weight loss should stop as the energy-losing glycosuria is abolished. Further investigation was thus necessary and this lady was found to have a carcinoma of the tail of her pancreas. Carcinoma of the pancreas can present as an apparent acute onset of diabetes and it is therefore important to think of secondary causes at the time of diagnosis.

Endocrine disease
The secondary endocrine causes involve excess endogenous production of hormones which are insulin antagonists (Box 1.1, p. 17). In acromegaly, growth hormone is secreted in excess by the pituitary gland.

In Cushing's syndrome, the adrenal cortex makes excess cortisol due either to a primary tumour within the adrenal gland or to excess ACTH production.

In phaeochromocytoma there is excess secretion of adrenaline or noradrenaline by a tumour of the adrenal medulla or sympathetic plexus.

Hypertension is seen in acromegaly, Cushing's syndrome and phaeochromocytoma and commonly accompanies NIDDM. When faced with an obese, hypertensive patient with an elevated blood glucose it is important to consider the possibility of an underlying endocrine disorder before accepting a diagnosis of NIDDM.

The exceedingly rare glucagonoma results in diabetes because glucagon also antagonises insulin.

Gestational diabetes occurs in about 4% of normal pregnancies and is due to the insulin-antagonising effects of placental steroids and human placental lactogen. Some women with gestational diabetes may need insulin treatment towards the end of pregnancy. Postnatally the diabetes goes into remission but these women will enter the 'at risk' category for developing NIDDM in later years (Ch. 2).

Drug therapy
The thiazide diuretics which are commonly used to treat essential hypertension have a blood glucose-raising effect by their inhibitory action on insulin secretion. Other drugs such as corticosteroids, e.g. prednisolone, also make tissues relatively resistant to the effects of insulin and thus unmask diabetes (Ch. 4).

Genetic syndromes

The genetic syndromes in Table 1.1 are rare but can be associated with diabetes mellitus although the mechanisms are unknown. The syndrome comprising diabetes insipidus, diabetes mellitus, optic atrophy and deafness (DIDMOAD) is a well recognised entity which can present with varying clinical features of the syndrome. Acanthosis nigricans, a rare skin condition sometimes associated with hirsutism and polycystic ovaries, is associated with a very insulin-resistant type of diabetes.

Incidence and prevalence

The incidence of a disease is the number of new cases arising each year. The prevalence is the number of people with a disease in the population at any one time. The incidence of diabetes varies from country to country and area to area within countries.

In the UK the prevalence of diabetes (both IDDM and NIDDM) is between 1 and 2% of the whole population.

Insulin-dependent diabetes

The incidence of IDDM in persons aged below 18 years in 1992 in Scotland was 24 per 100 000 of the population, whereas in the Oxford region of England this was 16 per 100 000 (Green et al 1992). Within Europe the incidence of IDDM appears to increase as one travels North, with Finland having more than 40 new cases per 100 000. In contrast Japan has only 1 to 2 per 100 000 of the population (Atkinson & MacLaren 1994).

There are two peak incidences of IDDM: around 5 years of age and again between the ages of 11 and 13 years. There is also a variation in incidence throughout the year with more patients diagnosed in the autumn and winter months.

Non-insulin-dependent diabetes

With the more common NIDDM, accurate figures of the incidence are difficult to establish because of inconsistent diagnostic criteria. The prevalence is difficult to determine accurately because of the relatively large population of people with NIDDM who remain undiagnosed.

The prevalence of NIDDM varies from country to country and population to population. Some Polynesian islanders, such as those from Nauru, have a prevalence of 1540 per 100 000 (Zimmet et al 1990).

NIDDM becomes more common with increasing age, with around 50% of patients attending hospital diabetic clinics aged over 60 years.

Aetiology of diabetes

Insulin-dependent diabetes mellitus

There is good evidence that IDDM is an organ-specific autoimmune disease with affected persons born with the tendency to destroy their own insulin-producing beta cells in the islets of Langerhans. There clearly must also be some environmental trigger since twin studies have shown that in only around 40% of identical twin pairs does the other twin develop diabetes (Barnett et al 1981).

Modern science is continually expanding our knowledge of the basic genetic defect, the nature of the environmental agent and the immunopathological processes.

Genetic predisposition

The risk of developing IDDM is mainly conferred by the inheritance of genes relating to the major histocompatibility complex (MHC) on chromosome 6. Recent gene mapping studies have shown that another important gene conferring susceptibility to diabetes is on chromosome 11, near the genes for insulin and insulin-like growth factor. In total there are 20 independent chromosomal regions associated with the genetic predisposition to IDDM (Atkinson & MacLaren 1994).

The MHC was discovered when transplantation immunologists were trying to find out why recipients rejected donor organs. Sitting on the surface of all cells are protein molecules which allow the immune system to recognise cells as being 'self' or 'foreign'. It is now known that these immune-system-recognition molecules known as HLA exist in two classes.

Class I molecules are present on all nucleated cells and platelets. These proteins are recognised by specialised white blood cells known as CD8 (cytotoxic or suppressor) T lymphocytes. The main function of this type of T lymphocyte is to recognise antigens such as a virus but this requires the close association of the HLA class I molecule.

Class II molecules of the HLA-D series (HLA-DP, DQ and DR) are present on other cells (not platelets nor nucleated cells) and present antigens to CD4 (helper or inducer) T lymphoctes. These T helper cells recognise antigens on macrophages and B lymphocytes. The complex interaction of these processes triggers activation and proliferation of T lymphocytes.

The main susceptibility genotypes for IDDM are HLA-DR3 and DR4. Some HLA-DR subtypes such as HLA-DR11 and DR15 protect against the development of diabetes. The mode of action of these susceptibility genes is unclear. They may either control the immune response to a pancreatic islet beta cell autoantigen such that an overly vigorous response initiates damage to the beta cell, or the genes may control the presentation of the beta cell autoantigen such that the immune system fails to recognise the beta cell as self.

There is clearly much to learn about these genetic processes. Why do certain HLA types (HLA-DR3 and HLA-DR4) predispose to the development of IDDM and others (HLA-DR11 and HLA-DR15) protect? Why are offspring of fathers with IDDM three times more likely to develop diabetes than the offspring of mothers with IDDM (Warram et al 1984)?

Pathogenesis of IDDM

Insulinitis

By examining the pancreases of patients with long-standing IDDM, it has been shown that there is destruction of the insulin-secreting beta cells while other cells are preserved. Even when pancreases of newly diagnosed patients are examined, most are deficient in beta cells. In other words, the destruction is highly selective to the beta cells.

In newly diagnosed patients there are large numbers of inflammatory cells including CD4 and CD8 T lymphocytes, B lymphocytes and others surrounding the beta cell. This is referred to as insulinitis. This inflammatory process is commonly associated with the presence of cytoplasmic antibodies in the peripheral blood. These circulating antibodies are more likely to be a marker of the insulinitis rather than the cause. In people with IDDM, about 80% of the beta cells in the pancreas require to be destroyed by this autoimmune pathological process before the patient presents with the more common symptoms of polyuria and polydipsia.

Circulating autoantibodies

Much has been learned about the natural history of IDDM by studying siblings of people with diabetes over a long period of time. Autoantibodies to islet cell cytoplasm are found in the serum of 3–4% of these siblings whereas only 0.5% of the normal population have them. The risk of developing IDDM in these siblings is related to the titre of his or her islet cell autoantibody (Bonifacio et al 1990, Deschamps et al 1992).

Antibodies against insulin itself (insulin autoantibodies) are also found in the serum of about 50% of newly diagnosed people with IDDM. The presence of both islet cell cytoplasmic antibodies and insulin autoantibodies in a sibling confers far greater risk than only one or the other alone. Studies which have examined islet cell ability to produce insulin in these siblings sequentially have shown that it takes many years for clinical diabetes to develop from the first immunological insult.

Other islet cell antigens against which autoantibodies have been detected in people with IDDM are being increasingly identified. It is unclear whether these are directly involved in causing diabetes or whether destruction of the beta cell exposes the antigens within the cell to the immune system which then produces the autoantibodies. The autoantibodies would then be a secondary phenomenon and they would simply act as markers for the disease.

It is probable that the disordered immune response to an environmentally introduced viral protein sharing a similar structure to a beta cell protein is the basis of the pathological process. Coxsackievirus protein has a similar structure to one islet cell enzyme and seems a likely candidate.

Another possible environmental trigger may be a 'life event' such as bereavement in a close family member.

Prevention of IDDM

These observations are important as they allow real prospects of preventing IDDM. Those people predisposed to develop IDDM can be identified by genetic and immunological markers. Studies are now ongoing using differing agents such as nicotinamide and subcutaneous insulin to see if the development of IDDM can be prevented (Chase et al 1990, Keller et al 1993).

Non-insulin-dependent diabetes mellitus

There is no evidence whatsoever that NIDDM is an autoimmune process. Twin studies have shown almost 90% concordance for NIDDM. It is more common in certain racial group such as Pima Indians and is much more likely to be a predominantly inherited condition (Knowler et al 1981). The genetic mechanisms have however proved elusive.

Many patients with NIDDM also have associated obesity. Despite the tendency to obesity being partly hereditary, its development is mainly related to environmental factors such as the enormous availability of food in developed nations and the cultural factors which make food such an important factor in physical and psychological well-being. It has been shown that individuals from fairly primitive societies, where the incidence of diabetes is low, who then move to societies where food is too readily available, often progress to develop diabetes (Mather 1991).

More recent epidemiological research has shown that patients developing NIDDM in later life were small babies at birth, suggesting that some intrauterine factor(s) might be important in determining susceptibility (Hales et al 1991).

Pathogenesis of NIDDM

There are three basic metabolic abnormalities in NIDDM. These are:

- insulin resistance
- impaired insulin secretion
- increased hepatic glucose production.

The sequence of events is shown in Figure 1.1.

Insulin resistance

The first step in developing NIDDM is probably a defect in the action of insulin resulting in impaired glucose uptake by the cells. To compensate for this and to maintain normal blood glucose levels there is a resulting increase in beta cell insulin secretion with consequent hyperinsulinaemia (Fig. 1.1). Over a number of years this continues with insulin-secreting beta cells working very hard to maintain a normal blood glucose.

As these overworked beta cells fail to keep pace with the insulin production required to maintain euglycaemia, impaired carbohydrate tolerance develops. Overt diabetes then follows, signalling that the beta cells are failing.

There is some evidence that this ineffectiveness of insulin action is inherited, and this is being actively investigated at present.

The insulin receptor on the cell surface binds circulating insulin (Fig. 1.2). This receptor is made up of two extracellular alpha

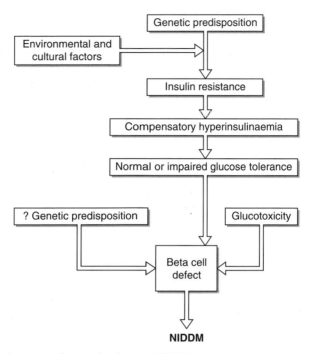

Fig. 1.1 Sequence of events leading to NIDDM.

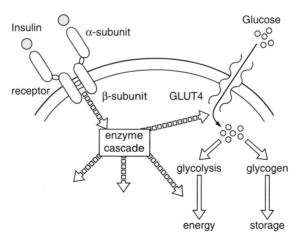

Fig. 1.2 The insulin receptor and its actions.

subunits which bind insulin and are connected through the cell membrane into the intracellular milieu with two beta subunits. Binding of insulin to the alpha units results in the beta subunits triggering a cascade of metabolic events which involve the enzyme tyrosine kinase and culminate in the entry of glucose into the cell and subsequent metabolic processing. The entry of glucose is mediated by GLUT4, a cell membrane glucose transporter. While abnormalities of this transporter might be expected to lead to NIDDM, none has yet been identified.

One of the important enzymes involved in the conversion of glucose into glycogen in muscle is glycogen synthase (GS), and abnormalities of this gene might also predispose to NIDDM. Further potential genetic defects might exist in proteins or enzymes functioning after insulin/insulin receptor binding and these remain to be elucidated.

There is no doubt that the state of insulin resistance is fairly dynamic and that certain physiological states influence this. Weight gain is known to increase insulin resistance and regular exercise to decrease it, and this explains why losing weight and exercise prescription are important measures in the treatment of NIDDM.

Impaired insulin secretion

This is the definitive event in the transition from insulin resistance to the diabetic state. As the beta cells fail and insulin levels fall, blood glucose rises and the person progresses from an insulin-resistant state to developing symptomatic diabetes. Whether the decline in beta cell function is genetically preprogrammed or whether this is acquired remains unclear.

Pathological studies in patients with NIDDM have shown a reduction in islet cell volume to 50–60% normal. Protein deposits including the polypeptide amylin are found around the islets and it is attractive to postulate that the presence of amylin might indicate an exhausted or prematurely aged islet.

In early NIDDM the basal insulin levels are normal or even increased but appear inappropriately low for the raised blood glucose. The immediate insulin response post-prandially is impaired and as blood glucose rises this in turn leads to further impairment. It appears as if higher glucose levels blunt subsequent insulin secretion—this is termed glucotoxicity. This glucotoxicity probably explains why so many NIDDM patients with acute symptoms of hyperglycaemia can respond fairly dramatically to the immediate removal or reduction of simple sugars in their diet. The rapid fall in blood glucose induced by dietary measures increases insulin secretion, which in turn helps to reduce the blood glucose still further.

Increased hepatic glucose output

In the pathogenesis of NIDDM there is reduced muscle and adipose cell glucose uptake as well as excessive glucose output from the liver. The liver can generate glucose from fat and protein (gluconeogenesis) and this process is under the influence of insulin. The mechanisms involved are poorly understood but reduced insulin in portal venous blood is important. The overall result is enhanced gluconeogenesis and hence hyperglycaemia.

Insulin and its actions

The hormone insulin is a 51 amino acid peptide secreted by the beta cells of the islets of Langerhans. The insulin gene is situated on the short arm of chromosome 11 and controls the formation of a large insulin precursor molecule called preproinsulin. In the cytoplasm of the beta cell, preproinsulin is cleaved by enzymes to form proinsulin which in turn is cloven by a peptidase enzyme to form insulin and C-Peptide. The insulin molecule (Fig. 1.3) consists of an A-chain (21 amino acids) and a B-chain (30 amino acids). Three disulphide bridges link the structure.

In patients with diabetes the measurement of C-Peptide (Connecting-Peptide) in plasma or urine allows the endogenous insulin secretory

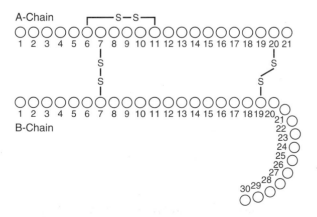

Fig. 1.3 The structure of insulin.

status of the beta cells to be assessed. This is sometimes measured in patients who are on insulin therapy to determine how much insulin their own pancreas is still producing.

The release of insulin from the beta cell can be stimulated by many factors including glucose, amino acids and sulphonylureas. Glucose enters the beta cell and is probably metabolised there in order to stimulate insulin release.

Other agents can increase insulin release. These include the neighbouring paracrine hormone glucagon from the alpha cells. Another hormone called gastric inhibitory polypeptide (GIP) also stimulates insulin release. This hormone is released when carbohydrate is eaten. It probably also explains why ingested glucose is a much more potent stimulus of insulin release than intravenous glucose. This also accounts for why the oral glucose tolerance test as opposed to the intravenous tolerance test is used for diagnostic purposes in NIDDM.

Glucose is absorbed from the small intestine and enters the portal vein. Most of the glucose then passes into the systemic circulation. The rise in blood glucose and GIP following a meal stimulates insulin release. Insulin then promotes glucose uptake from the circulation into fat and muscle cells and enhances the production of glycogen in liver and muscle. It increases amino acid uptake and protein synthesis in the tissues as well as preventing protein breakdown (Fig. 1.4).

The increased insulin also inhibits both the breakdown of protein to amino acids and triglycerides to free fatty acids and glycerol (Fig. 1.4).

When insulin has done its work, driving the higher blood glucose out of the circulation into the tissues after a meal, its production wanes and the blood glucose levels are then maintained by the finely tuned liver production of glucose.

In the fasting state, insulin levels fall. The fall in insulin levels allows the breakdown of fat and proteins to occur. The fatty acids provide the main fuel for muscles, leaving glucose free to fuel the brain. The low insulin concentrations are enough to limit ketone body formation and the normal buffering capacity of the blood prevents acidosis.

Diabetic ketoacidosis

In the pathological state of insulin deficiency there is an increased liver output of glucose from two sources. Glycogen is metabolised to

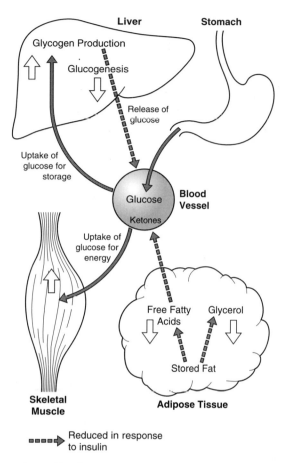

Fig. 1.4 The actions of insulin.

glucose and glucose is also formed (gluconeogenesis) from a combination of the breakdown products of fatty acids and amino acids (Fig. 1.4). In addition the lack of insulin results in less glucose being taken up by the peripheral tissues such as muscle. Blood glucose thus rises, overcoming the renal threshold for glucose with resulting glycosuria. The resulting osmotic diuresis is responsible for the symptoms of polyuria, nocturia and polydipsia in uncontrolled diabetes.

In addition fat and protein breakdown is quite unrestrained with consequent weight loss. Fatty acid levels rise very high, which in turn causes the liver to increase ketone body production. Ketone levels eventually overwhelm the acid buffering capacity of the blood with the development of ketoacidosis.

The combination of uncontrolled diabetes and acidosis with resultant circulatory collapse and clouded consciousness makes this a medical emergency which only intravenous fluids and insulin can reverse. Death can occur from diabetic ketoacidosis, although this is rare.

Hyperosmolar non-ketotic coma (HONK)

In a patient with HONK there is a relative, rather than complete, lack of insulin. This differentiates it from diabetic ketoacidosis. Here there is insufficient insulin production to prevent a rise in blood glucose yet there is just enough to prevent ketone body production. Hence ketonuria is not a feature.

Case Study 1.3

A 75-year-old woman is found lying on the floor by her home help who visits once per week. The woman is semiconscious and unable to give an account of what has happened to her. Her home help had found her rather tired and lethargic when she had called the previous week and on reflection states that the woman may have been drinking more fluid than normal. The woman is transferred immediately to hospital where she is found to be mildly hypothermic and clinically dehydrated. Her feet are mottled and the peripheral pulses are poor. Initial biochemistry confirms a dehydrated state with urea 22.5 mmol/l and creatinine 200 micromol/l. Her blood glucose is found to be 52 mmol/l!

HONK usually occurs in people with NIDDM. Patients may be undiagnosed as having NIDDM. The elderly, who are at most risk of HONK, failing to recognise the significance of their symptoms may become slowly unwell over a prolonged period. This can result in the blood glucose rising to very high levels (often >50 mmol/l) which causes a rise in plasma osmolality and results in severe dehydration. This too is a medical emergency. Treatment is by slow intravenous fluids and insulin to gradually correct the blood glucose level and avoid the added complication of cerebral oedema. When restored to good health, the patient is managed as the patient with NIDDM. Injected insulin is not usually necessary, suggesting that glucotoxicity may have played a role in the beta cell failure.

There is a high mortality rate associated with HONK due to the fact that patients may be comatose before they are discovered by relatives or friends. The dehydration reduces the circulation to the periphery and increases blood viscosity. Thrombosis of the arteries to the lower limbs is common and often contributes to the high mortality.

The counter-regulatory hormones

In both types of metabolic decompensation, DKA and HONK, it is important to recognise the actions of the hormones which oppose the action of insulin (Box 1.1).

Glucagon and catecholamines modulate beta cell insulin secretion. By increasing blood glucose levels they protect against hypoglycaemia and ensure fuel supplies to vital organs during stress. However in the stressful situations of DKA or HONK their actions are inappropriate and result in raising blood glucose to even greater levels.

The clinical differences between insulin-dependent and non-insulin-dependent diabetes

Age of onset

Patients with newly diagnosed IDDM are usually children or young adults but IDDM can be diagnosed at any age. NIDDM tends to present in patients over the age of 40 years. However, increasing numbers of patients are being identified at a younger age as awareness of NIDDM by patients and health care professionals improves.

Sex

IDDM is slightly more common in males, there being less sex bias in NIDDM.

Past medical history

Patients with IDDM have usually been very healthy before the development of diabetes. It is not uncommon however to find a history of hypertension and/or vascular disease in patients with NIDDM.

Box 1.1	Hormones which are antagonistic to the action of insulin	
• growth hormone	• catecholamines
• cortisol	• glucagon
• adrenaline	• placental steroids
• noradrenaline	• placental lactogen

Family history

Sometimes a family history of diabetes is seen in patients presenting with IDDM but this is more common in patients developing NIDDM.

Presentation

Patients with IDDM usually present with classical symptoms of polydipsia, polyuria, weight loss and tiredness. They may present with diabetic ketoacidosis.

Patients with NIDDM may also present with classical symptoms but never develop ketoacidosis. They more often present with symptoms associated with mild elevation of blood and urinary glucose—balanitis or vulvitis, blurred vision or leg cramps. NIDDM is more commonly diagnosed by the finding of glycosuria or hyperglycaemia in the course of assessment of other medical conditions or during routine screening tests. It is not uncommon for people with NIDDM to present with an established complication of diabetes such as background retinopathy during routine eye screening, or with an infected neuropathic foot ulcer.

Weight

Patients with IDDM have commonly lost weight at diagnosis, but not always. Many patients with NIDDM have coexistent obesity at diagnosis and it is not uncommon for some to claim recent great success in losing weight. This is of course due to the amount of energy lost in persisting glycosuria.

Urinalysis

Patients who present with classical symptoms of diabetes mellitus will have glycosuria. Ketonuria will be evident if presentation is with ketoacidosis. Most people with newly diagnosed IDDM will have significant ketonuria. Some people presenting with NIDDM can have small or moderate amounts of ketonuria. If this occurs it is usually because the person has reduced his/her calorie intake for whatever reason.

Sometimes, despite these clinical differences, it is difficult to tell if patients have IDDM or NIDDM. This may not matter too much in the sense that initial treatments may not differ. However, it may be crucial in some individuals to know if they are likely to require insulin treatment because this might have serious implications in relation to employment, insurance and driving (Ch. 10).

Summary

Diabetes mellitus is a chronic condition classified into two main types—insulin-dependent and non-insulin-dependent. IDDM is an autoimmune condition. Recent research has demonstrated defects in immunity which result in this condition. NIDDM is primarily an inherited disorder characterised by peripheral resistance to insulin with subsequent exhaustion of the pancreas's ability to secrete insulin.

Diabetes mellitus results in irreversible tissue damage and is a major source of morbidity and mortality within the population.

REFERENCES

Atkinson M A, MacLaren N K 1994 The pathogenesis of insulin dependent diabetes. New England Journal of Medicine 331:1428–1436
Barnett A H, Eff C, Leslie R D G, Pike D A 1981 Diabetes in identical twins: a study of 200 pairs. Diabetologia 20:87–93
Bliss M 1983 The discovery of insulin. Paul Harris Publishing, Edinburgh
Bonifacio E, Bingley P J, Shattock M, Dean B M, Dunger D, Gale E A M, Bottazzo G F 1990 Quantification of islet-cell antibodies and prediction of insulin-dependent diabetes. Lancet 335:147–149
Chase H P, Butler-Simon N, Garg S, McDuffie M, Hoops S L, O'Brien D 1990 A trial of nicotinamide in newly diagnosed patients with type 1 (insulin-dependent) diabetes mellitus. Diabetologia 33:444–446
Department of Health and British Diabetic Association 1995 St Vincent Task Force for Diabetes final report. BDA, London
Deschamps I, Boitard C, Hors J, Busson M, Marcelli-Borge A, Mogenat A, Robert J J 1992 Life table analysis of the risk of type 1 (insulin-dependent) diabetes mellitus in siblings according to islet cell antibodies and HLA markers: an 8 year prospective study. Diabetologia 35:951–957
Green A, Gale E A M, Patterson C C 1992 Incidence of childhood-onset diabetes mellitus: the EURODIAB ACE Study. Lancet 339:905–909
Hales C , Barker D J P, Clark P M S, Cox L J, Fall C, Osmond C, Winter P D 1991 Fetal and infant growth and impaired glucose tolerance at age 64 years. British Medical Journal 303:1019–1022
Keller R J, Eisenbarth G S, Jackson R A 1993 Insulin prophylaxis in individuals at risk of type 1 diabetes. Lancet 341:927–928
Knowler W C, Pettit D J, Bennett P H, Savage P I 1981 Diabetes incidence in Pima Indians: contributions of obesity and parental diabetes. American Journal of Epidemiology 113:144–156
Mather H M 1991 Diabetes mellitus in ethnic communities in the UK. In: Pickup J C, Williams G (eds) Textbook of diabetes. Blackwell Scientific, Oxford
Tattersall R B 1991 Maturity-Onset Diabetes of the Young. In: Pickup J C, Williams G (eds) Textbook of diabetes. Blackwell Scientific, Oxford
Warram J H, Krolewski A S, Gottlieb M S, Kahn C R 1984 Differences in risk of insulin-dependent diabetes in offspring of diabetic mothers and diabetic fathers. New England Journal of Medicine 311:149–152
Zimmet P, Dowse G, Finch C, Serjeantson S, King H 1990 The epidemiology and natural history of NIDDM—lessons to be learnt from the South Pacific. Diabetes/Metabolism Reviews 6:91–124

Diagnosis and screening for diabetes

Joan McDowell

2

INTRODUCTION

Most doctors and nurses would have no difficulties in diagnosing diabetes in the patient who presents with the classic symptoms of polyuria, polydipsia, weight loss and tiredness. In such patients the diagnosis is easily confirmed by a clearly elevated blood glucose level.

However, diagnosing non-insulin-dependent diabetes mellitus (NIDDM) is often more difficult since the onset is very gradual and diabetes may be present several years before the patient presents with any clinical symptoms (Harris et al 1992). The diagnosis of NIDDM often occurs by chance with the finding of glycosuria in a patient presenting with another medical problem or during a health screen. Sometimes patients may be diagnosed through screening programmes specifically for diabetes. The renal threshold for glucose rises with age. In the older patient, above 40 years, this means that there will be no glycosuria until the blood glucose level is significantly raised. Since glycosuria acts as an osmotic diuretic so it is responsible for the more common symptoms of polyuria and polydipsia.

The prevalence of diabetes within the United Kingdom (UK) is between 1 and 2%. Within the UK there are approximately 750 000 diabetics. As ageing is associated with a deterioration in glucose tolerance so the prevalence in the population rises to 5% or greater of those above 65 years (Peters & Davidson 1992). NIDDM accounts for 80% of all diabetes in the UK. This means that in a general practice of 2500 patients there will be on average about 36 diabetic patients of whom approximately 29 will have NIDDM and 7 will have insulin-dependent diabetes mellitus (IDDM). In addition it is estimated that 0.5% of the population have undiagnosed diabetes and hence within the general practice there would be a further 12 patients who have as yet undiagnosed diabetes.

Is there any value in diagnosing NIDDM before there are clinical symptoms? Undiagnosed diabetes is not a benign condition (Harris et al 1992). During the prediagnostic years, the unrecognised diabetes can result in complications developing and progressing. It is recognised that mortality rates are higher in the diabetic and undiagnosed diabetic population than in the nondiabetic population (Jarrett & Shipley 1988). Hence it would seem logical to diagnose diabetes before the patient develops diabetic complications or dies from associated vascular disease.

The undiagnosed diabetic usually presents in general practice with other associated medical conditions. Community nurses attending the elderly should be alert to the possibility of undiagnosed diabetes hindering a patient's anticipated recovery: for example, the slow-to-heal leg ulcer. Likewise General Practitioners and community nurses attending patients with a sore toe, vaginal or penile thrush, blurred vision, boils and carbuncles or complaints of weight loss must be proactive in their role to assist in the early detection of diabetes. Hence the presentation is varied and the onset of diabetic symptoms is insidious.

The Primary Health Care Team (PHCT) should be aware of the risk factors for developing NIDDM which are frequently associated with undiagnosed diabetes (Box 2.1). It is well recognised that there is a higher prevalence rate of NIDDM in all migrant Indo-Asian groups, i.e. those who migrate from a rural environment to an affluent, urban area (Roshan 1993). These risk factors are only pertinent to the patient with NIDDM. The aetiology of the patient with IDDM is described in Chapter 1.

Box 2.1   Risk factors for developing NIDDM

- family history of NIDDM
- obesity with a body mass index in excess of 25
- increasing age
- hypertension or significant hyperlipidaemia
- non-European race now resident within the UK
- gestational diabetes
- impaired glucose tolerance

DIAGNOSING DIABETES

The diagnosing of diabetes is clear where there are clinical symptoms and an unequivocal elevated blood glucose. Patients with symptoms and a random plasma glucose of 11.1 mmol/l or above or a fasting plasma glucose of 7.8 mmol/l or above are diabetic as defined by the World Health Organization (WHO 1985). Similarly it is easy to identify patients who are clearly not diabetic by finding a random plasma glucose below 5.5 mmol/l. The problem frequently arises in the community when a patient is found to have glucose levels between these extremes and does not complain of any of the usual signs and symptoms of diabetes.

Case Study 2.1

A 55-year-old woman attending the well woman clinic is found to have a glycosuria. A random plasma glucose is 10.8 mmol/l. On questioning she admits to nocturnal polyuria for a year which she had attributed to her age and her daily fluid intake. She does not complain of polydipsia but does enjoy drinking several cups of tea a day. She has had no weight loss within the previous year but admits to feeling tired. Her clinical symptoms are vague and not diagnostic of diabetes on this basis alone.

A careful history is taken to ascertain if this woman is taking any drugs, e.g. steroids or thiazide diuretics, which may reveal an underlying diabetic state. It is important to enquire into the health of her family as a family history of NIDDM predisposes this woman towards the same.

A random plasma glucose equal to or exceeding 11.1 mmol/l is usually indicative of diabetes although a diagnosis should not be made on the basis of only one abnormal finding in the absence of clinical symptoms (WHO 1985). In the asymptomatic patient two samples equal to or exceeding 11.1 mmol/l are required to confirm the diagnosis. Alternatively a random fasting plasma glucose equal to or exceeding 7.8 mmol/l on two occasions is confirmation of diabetes. Because this woman does not have a strong clinical presentation of diabetes and her random blood glucose test is equivocal, she would be advised to attend the surgery for an oral glucose tolerance test.

THE ORAL GLUCOSE TOLERANCE TEST (OGTT)

This test remains the definitive standard for diagnosing diabetes. Concerns are expressed regarding its poor reproducibility and the fact that it is subject to a wide variety of influences (Yudkin et al 1990). There are several factors which influence its reproducibility (Box 2.2). Despite the limitations of the OGTT it is still recommended if there is any doubt about the diagnosis (Bennett 1991). As a test however it is time-consuming for the patient, is rather unpleasant and may be quite inconvenient for both patient and staff.

It should be remembered that the OGTT is only conducted where there is an equivocal blood glucose result in the absence of any symptoms. It is usually performed within general practice; those hospitals who administer the test do so on an out-patient basis. Educating the patient prior to the test is essential to achieve some standardisation of the test. This is usually done by nursing staff and may be reinforced by literature. It is important that the patient knows who to contact with any queries regarding the test as it can be seen that many factors can influence the result.

Box 2.2   Factors which influence the OGTT

- prolonged bed rest
- restricting diet prior to the test
- the length of time in a true fast prior to the test
- any intercurrent illness
- drugs which the patient may be taking
- smoking during the test

Procedure

The test should be postponed if the patient is unwell or has required a prolonged period of bedrest prior to the test. The patient should consume their normal diet for three days before the test. It is therefore important not to commence the patient on a diabetic diet prior to the OGTT. The patient should fast overnight for 10–16 hours prior to the test. Water may be drunk during the fast. The OGTT should be performed in the morning and the patient advised not to smoke immediately prior to or during the test. The nurse responsible for the OGTT should record any factor which may influence the interpretation of the results, e.g. medications, mild infection (Box 2.3).

A sample for blood glucose estimation is taken when the patient is fasting. The patient is then advised to drink 75 g glucose diluted in warm water. This is usually palatable in the form of Lucozade. The amount of Lucozade is 400 ml, as 100 ml of Lucozade gives 18.7 g glucose. Therefore 400 ml gives 74.8 g glucose, which is as near equivalent to 75 g as possible. The patient should drink this within 5 minutes. A further blood glucose estimation is then taken 2 hours after the glucose load.

After the test a return appointment should be made to discuss the results, and the patient goes home. There is no particular aftercare required and the patient should be advised to live their life as normal until the return visit.

Interpreting the results

The WHO criteria for diagnosing diabetes have been developed over many years of research both in the UK and the United States of

---

Box 2.3   Checklist prior to administering the OGTT

- Does the patient feel well? If not, then record feelings in case notes.
- Has the patient been mobile according to his/her norms within the previous three days?
- Has the patient been consuming their normal diet for the previous three days? If not, then record alterations to diet.
- Ask the patient when he/she last ate and record the date and time.
- Ask the patient if he/she smokes. If so, then record the date and time of the last cigarette.
- Record any medications which the patient is taking.

America. Through these studies it was found that people who had a glucose level equal to or above 11.1 mmol/l two hours after a glucose challenge were at greatest risk of developing complications of diabetes, primarily retinopathy (Harris 1993). From these results the undernoted levels are derived (Table 2.1, WHO 1985).

In considering case study 2.1, there are four possible results which this woman could have.

Should none of her glucose samples exceed the levels in Table 2.1, then she does not have diabetes. Alternatively, if her plasma glucose levels exceed those in Table 2.1 then she has diabetes. Her management would then be as detailed in the succeeding chapters.

What if only one of her results was abnormal? Take for example a fasting plasma glucose of 6.0 mmol/l but a 2-hour plasma glucose of 12.1 mmol/l. The second result is clearly within the diabetic range; however, this woman does not have strong clinical symptoms. In this instance it would be desirable to wait until a second result was achieved which was also clearly within the diabetic range. The second result may be obtained from a random sample or repeat OGTT.

The last scenario is where this woman's results are equivocal. Her fasting plasma glucose could be normal or elevated but her 2-hour plasma glucose is 10.6 mmol/l. This is not within the diabetic range but is clearly an elevated result. This patient then has what is known as 'impaired glucose tolerance', and this is discussed below.

It is important when interpreting any glucose results that the person reading them knows whether the sample is on whole blood or plasma, venous or capillary, and interprets the results accordingly. Within the community it is usual for venous plasma samples to be collected.

Table 2.1 The diagnosis of diabetes after an OGTT. The patient has diabetes mellitus if his/her blood glucose result is greater than the levels indicated below 2 hours after 75 g glucose load

Glucose concentration (mmol/l)

Patient state	Whole blood		Plasma	
	Venous	Capillary	Venous	Capillary
Fasting	>6.7	>6.7	>7.8	>7.8
2 hours after 75 g glucose load	>10.0	>11.1	>11.1	>12.1

In some general practices there is a move towards taking a fasting blood glucose instead of undertaking a full OGTT. While this is not diagnostic for those who are asymptomatic it may be used as a screening test for diabetes and will be discussed under that heading.

IMPAIRED GLUCOSE TOLERANCE (IGT)

The state of IGT is unstable and patients may progress to diabetes or return to normal glucose tolerance. The numbers who revert to normal glucose tolerance vary considerably between 28 and 67% (Yudkin et al 1990). In clinical practice, does the diagnosing of IGT matter to the patient?

There is no doubt that IGT has very important clinical implications. IGT carries an increased risk of macrovascular disease, e.g. stroke and coronary heart disease (Jarrett & Shipley 1988). Therefore if a person is identified as having IGT they should be screened for other risk factors, e.g. smoking, obesity, lack of exercise, hypertension and hyperlipidaemia and thereafter encouraged to make the necessary lifestyle changes. It is recommended that as IGT is a risk factor for developing diabetes then patients with IGT should be screened every 3 years for diabetes (Paterson 1993).

The diagnosis of IGT is made on the glucose samples following an OGTT as detailed in Table 2.2 (WHO 1985).

SCREENING PROGRAMMES FOR DIABETES

How does one detect the large number of people with undiagnosed diabetes? Perhaps the answer is in screening programmes. The

Table 2.2 The diagnosis of impaired glucose tolerance after an OGTT. Consider the results below 2 hours after 75 g glucose load. The patient has IGT if his/her result lies within this range

Glucose concentration (mmol/l)				
Patient state	Whole blood		Plasma	
	Venous	Capillary	Venous	Capillary
Fasting	<6.7	<6.7	<7.8	<7.8
2 hours after 75 g glucose load	6.7–10.0	7.8–11.1	7.8–11.1	8.9–12.2

concept of screening is not new for community care as there has been a great increase in such clinics in general practice over recent years. A screening programme can only be effective if it meets certain criteria: sufficient people within the population who have the disease, clear benefits to the people from its early diagnosis, and a reliable test to screen for the disease.

NIDDM would appear to be sufficiently prevalent to warrant screening as it is estimated that there are approximately 300 000 undiagnosed NIDDM patients within the UK. Under the age of 40 years NIDDM is rare and therefore there is no value in screening this age group. As stated above, patients may have had NIDDM for many years before the diagnosis is made and patients may present with already well-establshed diabetic complications. There is increasing evidence that treating diabetes may prevent or delay the development of long term complications (The DCCT Research Group 1993). It would therefore appear likely that early diagnosis would be beneficial. These benefits are not just from the patient's perspective but also from that of the providers of health care as the treatment of diabetic complications has a significant impact on health resources.

There is also little benefit in screening for IDDM as those patients are quickly identified within a matter of days or weeks.

Identifying a reliable screening test for diabetes is much more difficult and will be discussed later in this chapter.

Venue for screening

Health screening can take place in a variety of settings in which community nurses may be involved. Local fairs and mobile health caravans often offer people health checks for blood pressure, weight, diet assessment, etc., and may form a basis for screening for diabetes as well. In this particular setting it is important that those doing the screening have adequate knowledge of how to screen for diabetes, the equipment being used, the interpretation of the result and the follow up advice essential for those identified as requiring further investigation. Any member of the Health Care Team may be requested to attend such local fairs. It is important that the individual team member recognises their own limitations within such a setting.

Community nurses routinely undertake screening by urinalysis of all new patients who are admitted to their case load. From the under-noted discussion on which tests are most suitable and by nature of the number of patients involved, the detection rate for diabetes is bound to be small. However, it does remain the screening test of choice for community nurses.

Nurses undertaking more structured screening must be adequately trained and demonstrate competence in knowledge and skills necessary for undertaking the tests.

Each PHCT is encouraged to develop their own protocols for screening. The decision may be made to target certain people.

Targeting for screening

In considering the difficulties in screening for diabetes it would seem reasonable that only those considered to be at risk of developing diabetes should be screened. By the rationalisation of screening to target populations, a more cost-effective use of resources is achieved.

To define this target population it is recommended that screening is restricted to those with risk factors (Box 2.1) and who are between 40 and 75 years of age (Paterson 1993). The PHCT may also decide to screen every new patient over the age of 40 years who joins the practice.

It is clearly obvious that the responsibility for screening for diabetes is with the PHCT. By incorporating this into other clinics it need not be an impossible task, an unnecessary burden on staff, nor a drain on resources. Any screening protocols however must be cost-effective and reach those people most at risk of developing diabetes.

Screening is therefore recommended within the general practice setting (Paterson 1993). The PHCT know the individual patients and their families. They are more able to counsel the patient and answer the patient's questions which may arise if a screening test is positive. The person being screened should be kept fully informed of the test being used and the result obtained. Each primary care team know their own resources and availability of staff for follow up. The management of the patient commences in general practice and it seems most appropriate that screening for diabetes should be based there too.

The choice of screening test used is decided by the PHCT who should formulate their own policy regarding this.

SCREENING TESTS FOR DIABETES

Any screening programme must use a simple test to discriminate between those who are likely to have the disease and those who are not. For a screening test to be widely acceptable it must be simple, cause little discomfort and be of minimal inconvenience to the person concerned. The benefits to the person of early diagnosis must be obvious before they consent to screening.

The British Diabetic Association (BDA) recommends that only three tests are considered for screening for diabetes. These are:

- a blood glucose 2 hours after a 75 g glucose load
- a fasting blood glucose
- post-prandial glycosuria (Paterson 1993).

These screening tests are not diagnostic of diabetes but rather indicative that further investigation is required.

There are various other tests available for screening which will be discussed in turn and the explanation given as to how the above three are the only recommended ones.

Urine testing

A urine test is easy to perform, is inexpensive and not too inconvenient for the patient. It may be the screening test of choice for community nurses when home visiting. It is one of the screening tests which is recommended by the BDA (Paterson 1993).

In the patient who is beginning to develop diabetes but who does not yet have overt clinical symptoms, glycosuria is more likely to occur following ingestion of food. For this reason, testing urine 2 hours after a large meal or a glucose load is more likely to identify a patient with diabetes compared to a fasting urine sample which may be negative for glucose. The BDA therefore does not recommend a fasting urine test for screening purposes.

As stated previously, the renal threshold for glucose rises with age. This means that any glycosuria in the older patient is likely to mean that there is a corresponding hyperglycaemia. The presence of glycosuria in the older patient will confidently detect diabetes. However, the raised renal threshold also means that some patients who have a mildly elevated blood glucose level will go undetected. This is because the mildly elevated blood glucose levels are insufficiently high to produce glycosuria. Hence a negative urine test does not imply the absence of diabetes.

Urine testing when positive will confidently identify the patient with diabetes. A positive screening test for glucose means that the patient should be referred to their GP for diagnosis of diabetes and future management. However when the test is negative, diabetes cannot be excluded with confidence and the test is therefore said to have a low sensitivity. This limits its usefulness as a screening test.

Recent government legislation recommends that general practitioners should screen all their patients between the ages of 16 and 75 years for glycosuria (Department of Health 1991). From the above it can be seen that this is a waste of resources due to the lack of accuracy of urine testing and the fact that the age range is too wide to detect NIDDM.

Blood testing

The fasting blood glucose is remarkably constant from day to day in both normal subjects and patients with NIDDM. A fasting blood glucose should be obtained after a fast of 10–16 hours (Bennett 1991). It is a useful test for screening but will inevitably miss those subjects with mild glucose intolerance whose hyperglycaemia only occurs after a glucose load. A fasting blood glucose test therefore has low sensitivity, missing some patients who do in fact have diabetes.

A fasting blood glucose however is fairly easy to acquire. The guidelines for interpreting the results are in Box 2.4. People with an equivocal result should be re-screened in 6–12 months.

A random blood glucose could be considered for diabetic screening. However as blood glucose levels fluctuate widely depending upon the time and content of the previous meal, this test is not recommended as a screening test.

While glycated haemoglobin tests are easy to obtain and are not dependent on recent food consumption they are unsatisfactory as screening tests because of the distribution overlap between diabetic

---

Box 2.4 Guidelines for interpreting the result after screening for diabetes using a fasting blood glucose sample (Paterson 1993)

- Plasma glucose <5.5 mmol/l or whole blood glucose <5.0 mmol/l is a negative screen.
- Plasma glucose 5.5–6.6 mmol/l or whole blood glucose 5.0–6.0 mmol/l is an equivocal result.
- Plasma glucose >6.6 mmol/l or whole blood glucose >6.0 mmol/l is a positive screening test.

and nondiabetic results. This means that they miss diagnosing people who do have diabetes. One problem is that different laboratories have different techniques for measuring glycated haemoglobins. It is therefore difficult to interpret and compare results between people, the laboratories and the techniques used. Although each laboratory will have its own range of normal results there is still an overlap between patients who have diabetes and those who do not. Inadequate standardisation, overlap of results and cost of the process do not make them good screening tests. The delay between taking the test and receiving a result also prohibits its use in a screening programme.

While WHO have identified the OGTT as the criterion for the diagnosis of diabetes, this test is time-consuming and inconvenient for the patient and costly to administer on a large scale. Therefore its use as a screening test for diabetes is questionable.

The modified OGTT can however be used as a screening test. Here the person being screened consumes a 75 g load of glucose and attends the surgery or screening centre for a blood glucose estimation 2 hours later. A fasting blood glucose is therefore not obtained. This unsupervised test clearly depends upon good patient cooperation and understanding of the need to attend exactly 120 minutes after consuming the glucose drink, having consumed no other food in the interim. The guidelines for interpreting the result are detailed in Box 2.5.

This 2-hour post-challenge test is probably the best screening test for diabetes. A negative result correctly identifies most people who do not have diabetes. The test is therefore said to have high specificity. However it is a more complex test, requires a highly motivated patient and may be expensive as part of a large screening programme.

Patient advice after a screening test

It is recommended that those with a positive screening test or equivocal result require a formal diagnosis to be made in line with

---

Box 2.5   Guidelines for interpreting the result after screening for diabetes using the modified OGTT (Paterson 1993)

Capillary plasma >8.8 mmol/l or capillary whole blood >8.0 mmol/l or venous plasma >8.0 mmol/l is a positive screening test.

the WHO criterion detailed above using a full OGTT (Paterson 1993). The person should be advised that the test has indicated that there is a possible rise in their blood glucose and that this should be investigated further. They should be instructed to make an appointment to attend their GP surgery at their earliest convenience and not to alter their diet in the meantime.

The effects on the person of the possibility of diabetes should not be underestimated. The nurse must be prepared to counsel such people to help alleviate their anxieties before a definite diagnosis is made. The screening for diabetes may result in people who feel well being told that in fact they are ill! This may have implications for their employment prospects, life insurance, driving licence, etc. It is therefore imperative that appropriate advice and counselling is offered to the person being screened at this stressful time. It is further recommended that those with a negative screening test and no risk factors for diabetes should be re-screened every 5 years. Those who have risk factors, e.g. family history of diabetes, Afro-Asian origin, should be screened every 3 years (Paterson 1993). However, within general practice these recommendations may be considered impossible and hence a decision may be made to develop a team policy to target certain age groups or ethnic minority groups for screening. The frequency of this screening programme will depend on resources within the PHCT.

PUBLIC AWARENESS OF DIABETES

Since diabetes is difficult to diagnose in the absence of clinical symptoms, difficult to screen for yet has debilitating effects on the patient, then perhaps increasing public awareness of the disease may increase the number of patients presenting earlier to their GP.

One recent study attempted to determine the impact of posters on the knowledge of the public on the symptoms of diabetes (Singh et al 1994). The posters chosen were predominantly in written form and were aimed to educate on the symptoms of diabetes. They also had a positive tone to them. It was hoped that this would avoid causing anxiety which could result in people not seeking help should they have the symptoms.

The results of this study confirmed an increase in the general public's awareness of the common symptoms of diabetes without intimidating them or causing undue anxiety. Furthermore the hypothesis that increasing the general public's knowledge about the symptoms of diabetes would lead to the early diagnosis of NIDDM was supported (Singh et al 1994). Hence it does compare competitively with other conventional screening methods.

As a potential form of early detection for NIDDM this area has to be researched further. Attempts by the BDA to secure financial support from the Department of Health for this purpose have been disappointing.

Community nurses may also be involved in setting up local campaigns with the purpose of increasing awareness of diabetes. In such a situation there must be adequate back-up resources for the potential influx of patients who wish to enquire about their health.

CONCLUSION

Diabetes has high morbidity and mortality rates. Particular concern is expressed regarding the diagnosing of those patients who are as yet unaware that they have the disease. This is due to the fact that they often present when they already have complications of the disease and early detection of diabetes may assist in the prevention of diabetic complications.

There are various tests available which can be used to diagnose diabetes, to screen for diabetes and to monitor diabetes (Ch. 7). It is important that the correct test is used for the correct purpose to facilitate the correct interpretation of the results.

All members of the PHCT have a role to play in the diagnosing of diabetes. Nurses have a particularly important role as they tend to spend more time with the patient and are more actively involved in the actual organisation of clinics. Being alert to the possibility of diabetes in the older patient and adopting the appropriate methods of screening or diagnosing diabetes can identify the newly diagnosed patient before the symptoms or complications are evident.

Increasing the knowledge of the general public regarding the symptoms of diabetes through poster campaigns is an effective way to persuade patients to self-select for further investigation for diabetes, but this method does require further research.

REFERENCES

Bennett P H 1991 Classification and diagnosis of diabetes mellitus and impaired glucose tolerance. In: Pickup J C, Williams G (eds) Textbook of diabetes. Blackwell Scientific, Oxford

The DCCT Research Group 1993 The effect of intensive treatment of diabetes on the development and progression of long-term complications in insulin-dependent diabetes mellitus. The New England Journal of Medicine 329:14:977–986

Department of Health 1991 The terms and conditions of service for doctors in general practice. Department of Health, London

Harris M 1993 Undiagnosed NIDDM: Clinical and public health issues. Diabetes Care 16:4:642–652

Harris M I, Klein R, Welborn T A, Knuiman M W 1992 Onset of NIDDM occurs at least 4–7 yr before clinical diagnosis. Diabetes Care 15:7:815–819

Jarrett R J, Shipley M J 1988 Type II (non-insulin dependent) diabetes mellitus and cardiovascular disease—putative association via common antecedents; further evidence from the Whitehall Study. Diabetologia 31:737–740

Paterson K R 1993 Population screening for diabetes mellitus. Diabetic Medicine 10:777–781

Peters A L, Davidson M B 1992 Ageing and diabetes. In: Alberti K G M M, De Fronzo R A, Keen H, Zimmer P (eds) International textbook of diabetes mellitus, Vol 2. John Wiley, Chichester

Roshan M 1993 Non-insulin-dependent diabetes in UK Indo-Asians. Diabetes in General Practice 3:3:27–29

Singh B M, Prescott J J W, Guy R, Walford S, Murphy M, Wise P H 1994 Effect of advertising on awareness of symptoms of diabetes among the general public: the British Diabetic Association Study. British Medical Journal 308:632–636

World Health Organization 1985 Technical Report Series No 727: Diabetes mellitus. World Health Organization, Geneva

Yudkin J S, Alberti K G M M, McLarty D G, Swai A B M 1990 Impaired glucose tolerance. British Medical Journal 301:397–402

Psychological care

Florence J. Brown

■ CONTENTS

INTRODUCTION

Diabetes has a major psychological and social impact on people's lives. The diagnosis of diabetes has major implications for the person involved and their family. The way people view their diagnosis of diabetes differs and this can affect the way in which they might look after themselves.

Coupled with this, life events such as bereavement or redundancy clearly affect diabetic control. Whilst diabetes can cause psychological and social problems—so psychological and social problems can upset diabetic control.

Community nurses are in a unique position to contribute high quality psychological care as an essential component of diabetes nursing. Their view of the patient's experience of living with diabetes on a day-to-day basis is uncluttered by the institutional elements of hospital care that often mask individuality. This chapter will explore some of the psycho-social difficulties of living with a life-long condition, the significance of major life events on diabetic control and how both can affect self-care practices. Methods of enhancing the delivery of psychological care with particular emphasis on defining the term 'counselling', the varying uses of counselling skills and the importance of integrating them into diabetes care will also be discussed.

THE PERSONAL MEANING OF HAVING DIABETES

Let us first undertake some self-analysis. Suppose you had just been diagnosed as having NIDDM. You may have been told that you are at a greater risk of heart attack or stroke and at an earlier age. You might already have some of the microvascular complications such as diabetic retinopathy or diabetic nephropathy, because apparently you had been diabetic for some years, but it had gone undiagnosed. You might also have other risk factors associated with diabetes and cardiovascular disease, such as hypertension, obesity, smoking or hyperlipidaemia. Receiving this information can be quite frightening, but how can one take such a disease seriously when there are often no symptoms? You might also have been told your diabetes was 'mild'!

Alternatively, what would distress you most about having IDDM? Would it be the injections or blood glucose monitoring or the restrictions on what and when you can eat? Or would it be hypoglycaemia and its risks, or the long-term complications of hyperglycaemia?

From the above, the diagnosis of diabetes, whether NIDDM or IDDM, will mean different things to different people. How people feel about having diabetes and what self-care practices they adopt will vary widely. The challenge in diabetes care is to acknowledge the patient's personal experience of living with diabetes and be aware that there may be unconscious influences at work which prevent healthy self-care practices. Ultimately people want to take good care of themselves but may be hindered by psycho-social issues (Rogers 1980). Examples of some of these unconscious influences are given later in the chapter.

Education is a major aspect of nursing the patient with diabetes and so it is important to consider some of the psychological elements of learning and behaviour change.

PSYCHOLOGICAL CARE AND DIABETES EDUCATION

How can the community nurse individualise patient education while attending to the patient's agenda, as well as her own? The community nurse must first consider the patient's personal and unique experience of living with diabetes and that its management impinges on every aspect of the patient's life (Brown, in press).

Traditionally diabetes education was seen as an information-giving exercise. The assumption was that once information was received, good self-care practices would follow. Take for example a patient who has failed to carry out blood glucose monitoring. One approach would be to assume that for some reason, he had not understood either the procedure, or the importance of doing the procedure. The teaching session could then be repeated with a demonstration of the procedure and the patient encouraged to practise the skill. The importance of blood glucose monitoring on a regular basis would be re-emphasised. However, there might be another reason for the patient's failure to comply: 'I can't bring myself to test my blood. Every time I think about it I feel angry about it, and about having diabetes. Why me? I don't need this. I've got enough on my plate, I'm not going to do it.'

Here the patient might ignore blood testing because he has not yet accepted his diabetes. Blood glucose monitoring reminds him physically that he has diabetes. He may want to deny his diabetes as a way of coping, and blood glucose monitoring would remind him, in an emotionally painful way, of his anger about having diabetes.

It is important to make diabetes education relevant on an individual level (Coles 1989). Information given about diabetes should be related to the patient's day-to-day life. In order to relate relevant information it is appropriate that community nurses should get to know their patient, understand the patient's lifestyle and be aware of their values in life (Ch. 10).

STRESS AND DIABETES

Major life events and daily hassles

Everyone has major life events from time to time. Life events can be graded according to how disruptive to one's life they are (Holmes & Rahe 1967). For example, death of a spouse, divorce or redundancy come near the top of the list for causing most disruption and stress (Box 3.1). Marriage and moving house come somewhere in the middle, and holidays and Christmas come closer to the bottom. On the other hand the accumulation of minor routine aspects of daily

---

Box 3.1   Life events in decreasing order of severity (Holmes & Rahe 1967)

Death of a partner
Separation or divorce
Death of close family member or friend
Personal injury or illness
Marriage
Dismissal from job
Marital reconciliation
Retirement
Change in health of family member
Pregnancy
Sex difficulties
New baby
Changes at work
Change in financial situation
Son or daughter leaving home
Outstanding personal achievement
Starting or leaving school
Trouble with boss
Moving house
Change in school
Going on holiday
Christmas

---

living, also called 'daily hassles', can result in the person feeling stressed (Shillitoe 1988, Holmes & Rahe 1967). Going through a major life event or daily hassles can produce certain degrees of stress which interfere with diabetes both physiologically and psychosocially.

What is stress?

It has been recently suggested that 'the essence of stress is the feeling of doubt about being able to cope ...' (Lancet 1994). The reasons why people feel they can or cannot cope are wide and varied. Some people cope with very major problems, others are unable to cope with apparently minor difficulties.

If people experience sustained stress, they may develop symptoms such as depression, agitation, apparently irrational anger, lethargy, anxiety, feeling muddled or irritability. Chronically tensed muscles can lead to general aches and pains including headache and there may be other symptoms such as indigestion, palpitations, diarrhoea, skin problems and loss of sex drive.

During times of stress, people find that their diabetes becomes more difficult to control. Most people find that their blood glucose seems to rise during stress, but others find that they alternate between hypoglycaemia and hyperglycaemia. This happens for two reasons. The first reason is a physiological response to stress which produces several stress hormones including adrenaline. These hormones work in opposition to the action of insulin and usually the blood glucose rises. Less commonly some people may become hypoglycaemic in response to stress and this mechanism is less well understood (Bradley & Cox 1978).

The second reason is that when people are experiencing stress, they try to find ways of alleviating the symptoms and blocking out the problems that are causing the stress. This is usually of a behavioural nature. Some people find that they eat more than usual or turn to more highly refined carbohydrate foods such as chocolate! Others may drink more alcohol than usual and smokers tend to smoke more cigarettes. Other people find that they lose their appetite when they are under stress and this may be another reason for hypoglycaemia at that time. These responses to stress are widespread but unfortunately can interfere with diabetic control.

GRIEF AND DIABETES

It is usual for people to experience a sense of loss in response to all sorts of situations, including someone dying, the break-up of a relationship, redundancy or retirement. Even the diagnosis of diabetes can involve grieving for the loss of health and lifestyle, or grieving can occur on the development of diabetic complications.

Grieving is well described as a staged process of coming to terms with the new situation. People experience a variety of reactions including denial, anger, bargaining, isolation and depression before acceptance (Kubler Ross 1990). It is a normal reaction and people vary in how long they take to come to terms with their loss.

Case Study 3.1

A woman in her late forties came to see the nurse because she knew her diabetes was 'out of control'. She wasn't eating well and she was either hypoglycaemic because she hadn't eaten sufficient or feeling tired and thirsty because she had eaten too much of the 'wrong' foods. When asked if there was anything else going on in her life that was causing her to overeat, she burst into tears and cried vigorously about the death of her father.

Initially it was thought that the woman's father had died within the last few days, but it transpired that he had died 9 months before. It was obvious that the woman had not made any progress in grieving for her father. On further questioning the reason became obvious. The woman's father had lived with her for 9 years. During that time the woman and her husband had never had a holiday, and they had finally decided to spend a week away on their own. The woman's father went to stay with his other daughter, but within 24 hours had died suddenly and unexpectedly. This resulted in the woman being consumed with guilt, believing that if she had been less selfish about going on holiday, her father would still be alive.

This woman required counselling for her grief before attempting to control her diabetes. During counselling sessions the woman had a conversation with her father, imagining that he was sitting in the empty chair opposite her. After she had expressed her sorrow and guilt about his death to him, she sat in the empty chair and pretended that she was her father and responded to what she had just said. 'He' reminded her that he had been very happy for her to go on holiday and had also been happy with the arrangement of staying with her sister. 'He' also mentioned that he had had a bad heart for a long time and that he might have died at any time; it was just so unfortunate that it had happened at that time when she was away.

When the 'conversation' had finished the woman said that she knew that what 'he' said was exactly what he would have said if he had been alive. This one session helped the woman to be rational about what had happened. This technique of counselling is called the Gestalt empty chair technique (Jones 1992). She subsequently stopped overeating, and her diabetic control improved. She also made dramatic progress in coming to terms with her father's death.

COPING STRATEGIES

People have different ways of coping with difficulties in their lives.

Unconscious strategies such as denial, obsessional behaviour and projection are employed to lessen the impact of living with diabetes.

Denial

It is a normal and protective response for some people to use 'switching off' or denial as a way of coping. Denial may be present at diagnosis and remain for several years afterwards. However, the presence of denial can also cause the person to be 'switched off' from good self-care practices (Anderson 1986). For example: 'I really don't think the diabetes is a problem. I have never felt better. I wonder if the doctor has made a mistake—I mean, I don't do as they ask me to do, and I am neither up nor down—what's the point in going to the clinic?'

Obsessional behaviour

Some people who experience a great deal of anxiety in relation to their diabetes find that they feel more in control if they are very precise about their self-care practices. They may monitor their blood and their urine more frequently than requested and document everything they have eaten. They are particularly aware of calorie and carbohydrate exchanges and try to make sense of differences in glycaemic levels in terms of their energy expenditure, diet, stress levels, etc. This sort of behaviour suggests that the patient may not have come to terms with the diagnosis: 'The doctor said that I could cut down my blood testing to two days a week instead of testing every day and he asked me to stop urine testing altogether. But I don't want to reduce my testing. I always like to know what is going on. I feel much safer if I am testing every day.'

Projection

The health care professional encourages patients to take responsibility for their diabetes. However, the patient with diabetes might believe that what happens to his diabetes, good or bad, is as a result of outside influences. He projects or places the responsibility of his diabetes onto others—doctors, nurses, relations or friends: 'I said to the doctor that the diet the dietitian has given me is completely unacceptable. I can't be eating one thing and my family eating another. The dietitian said that I should give my family the same diet as me, she said it was healthy for all of us, but I told her that the family wouldn't put up with that . . . anyway, it is far too expensive.'

In projecting responsibility onto others the patient is demonstrating an external locus of control.

The health locus of control model says that patients demonstrate internal locus of control when they believe that their health is their own responsibility. Having external locus of control means that the patient believes that his health is the responsibility of others and that what happens to him is a result of influences beyond his control (Becker 1974).

The issues of responsibility and making choices are components in psychological care and in the concept of patient empowerment.

PSYCHOLOGICAL CARE AND EMPOWERMENT

What is empowerment?

The concept of empowerment has been gathering momentum in health promotion literature over the last 10 years (Ewles & Simnet 1992, Tones et al 1990, WHO 1984): 'Health promotion is the process of enabling people to increase control over, and to improve, their health' (WHO 1984).

The concept suggests that people should be enabled to assume more control over those aspects of their lives which affect their health. Patients are expected to participate actively in health care and decision making (Table 3.1).

One self-empowerment model is considered in more detail. It takes into account knowledge and practical skills, self-efficacy, self-esteem, health beliefs and values and a repertoire of social skills including assertiveness (Tones 1991).

Empowerment in diabetes care

The notions of personal responsibility and active participation in diabetes care were described by R D Lawrence, a doctor with IDDM and one of the founding members of the British Diabetic Association (Lawrence 1935). However, the complexity of the concept of patient self-empowerment has only been in evidence more recently (Anderson 1995, Feste 1992, Funnell et al 1991). For patients to be self-empowered, knowledge, skills, attitudes and self-awareness are required. These are necessary to influence their own behaviour and that of others so that the quality of their lives can be improved (Funnell et al 1991, Tones 1991). To facilitate self-empowerment, health professionals

Table 3.1 Comparison of traditional and empowering educational models (Funnell et al 1991)

Traditional medical model	Empowering person-centred model
1. Diabetes is a physical illness.	1. Diabetes is a biopsycho-social condition.
2. Relationship of nurse and patient is authoritarian based on nurse expertise.	2. Relationship of nurse and patient is democratic and based on shared expertise.
3. Problems and learning needs are usually identified by nurse.	3. Problems and learning needs are usually identified by patient.
4. Nurse is viewed as problem solver and caregiver.	4. Patient is viewed as problem solver and caregiver, i.e., the nurse acts as a resource and both share responsibility for treatment and outcome.
5. Goal is compliance with recommendations. Behavioural strategies are used to increase compliance with recommended treatment. A lack of compliance is viewed as a failure of patient.	5. Goal is to enable patients to make informed choices. Behavioural strategies are used to help patients change behaviours of their choosing. A lack of goal achievement is viewed as feedback and used to modify goals and strategies.
6. Behaviour changes are externally motivated.	6. Behaviour changes are internally motivated.
7. Patient is powerless, nurse is powerful.	7. Patient and nurse are powerful.

need to change their own attitude and approach towards patients within the traditional medical model of diabetes consultation to a person-centred empowering model (Funnell et al 1991, and see Table 3.1). This can be achieved by the use of counselling skills in the consultation.

Knowledge and practical skills

The fundamental requirements for making informed choices are knowledge and skills. Participatory methods of diabetic education that are tailored to help the individual patient cope with day-to-day requirements are advocated (Shillitoe 1987). He goes on to emphasise the importance of watching what patients do in terms of practical skills. These include such things as actual preparation of meals or managing blood glucose levels and diet during actual exercise rather than talking about it. He argues that this kind of experiential education increases self-confidence and the ability to cope.

Self-efficacy

This is how much one believes one can influence, control or take charge of one's life (Bandura 1977). It includes the capacity to deal with social pressures. Self-efficacy describes the abilities or otherwise that a person has to effect control on one's life and is related to the kind of outcome from experiential education described above. If someone has an internal locus of control but does not have the skills to effect change or control, then that person might develop 'learned helplessness'. This '. . . refers to a psychological state of motivational loss, emotional disturbance, and cognitive impairment, which is induced in any person exposed repeatedly to an uncontrollable and unpleasant situation' (Dunn 1987).

Dunn gives an example of a young man who became aggressive and hostile following his inability to improve glycaemic control despite his best efforts over a number of weeks. The man became sullen, lost his enthusiasm and gave up blood glucose monitoring altogether. Eventually he was referred for psychological assessment because of developing reactive depression. Following consultation, Dunn outlines a more realistic programme of goals along with individualised educational support. This enabled the man to view his own personal situation with more insight and helped to alleviate his 'helplessness' and depression.

Self-esteem

This describes the thoughts and feelings a person has about him or herself based on how that person has been valued by others. 'It indicates the extent to which we believe ourselves to be significant, capable and worthy' (Stewart).

Self-esteem can change. Personal achievement or being in a good relationship can give someone a high self-esteem but if misfortune befalls or a significant relationship becomes difficult then that same person might develop a low self-esteem. Some people find it difficult to achieve even reasonable self-esteem if they come from a background of emotional deprivation.

Health beliefs

There are four important belief factors that determine whether or not an individual will follow the treatment recommended. These beliefs concern perceptions of

- the severity of the disorder
- vulnerability to the disorder
- the benefits of treatment
- the barriers to treatment (Becker 1974).

A patient's readiness to follow the treatment regimen is highly dependent on two aspects. The first aspect is the perceived desirability of avoiding the symptoms and the complications of the disorder. The second aspect is the belief that the health actions necessary will be effective but not too costly when compared to other valued aspects of the individual's lifestyle.

A specific health belief scale in relation to diabetes has been developed (Bradley et al 1984, Lewis et al 1990). The main purpose of the scales are to measure beliefs about diabetes and its complications in order to understand individual differences and preferences for treatment regimens and their efficacy. The scales measure perceived benefits of and barriers to treatment and perceived severity of and vulnerability to the complications of diabetes. Health beliefs have been cited as important components of empowerment (Feste 1992, Tones 1991).

Assertiveness

Assertiveness helps people communicate their rights and feelings more clearly and confidently. Sometimes people find it difficult to say 'No' and often find themselves agreeing to things that are detrimental to their health and well-being. This kind of response can leave people feeing angry and resentful. Some people feel they can only say 'No' if they have a 'good' excuse. Assertiveness does not mean being aggressive. Patients find asserting themselves with a health professional difficult especially if that health professional gives an air of expertise which may be difficult to disagree with.

The self-empowerment model is widely used in health promotion and is very relevant to diabetes care. However it does not mean that if a patient is self-empowered he is necessarily following the rules of diabetes self-management.

Case Study 3.2

A 49-year-old, intelligent and articulate sales manager has had IDDM for 30 years. He has most of the diabetic complications including diabetic nephropathy which required a kidney transplant 2 years previously, retinopathy and neuropathy. His blood glucose levels remain consistently high, although having developed complications, he might be expected to be highly motivated to improve his diabetic control, not least to protect his new kidney. Several education sessions fail to persuade him to adjust his insulin in a preventative way rather than in a crisis intervention way. When eventually he is asked at what levels he prefers his blood glucose to be, he explains that he would rather risk further deterioration in his complications than risk hypoglycaemia. For him, hypoglycaemia was an experience akin to a nightmare.

'I know that I am putting myself at risk in terms of worsening eye and kidney disease but I cannot put myself at risk of hypoglycaemia, I would never be able to relax. I don't get the warnings anymore, I would have to stop driving and then I would lose my job and maybe my home as a result. I know you regularly check the progress of my complications and so I have decided that this is how I must live my life.'

This man had made a choice, an informed choice, about his diabetic management.

The health care professionals often quote that the patient is the expert. However it would seem that the true meaning of empowerment is not always fully understood. Is a patient only an expert in his condition if he is adhering to the rules? If the patient has chosen to live his life in a certain way which might not be conducive to long-term good health, and if his choice is based on knowledge and not affected by emotional distress, has the health care team any right to contest that choice? The professional barrier comes if the health care team do not agree with that patient's choice and resort to other methods of coercing the patient into changing his behaviour. Methods such as threats of complications are actually unlikely to influence change and may ultimately have a negative outcome on the most precious tool of all—the professional/patient relationship.

Professionally it is difficult to accept that some patients might choose to lead a lifestyle not conducive to avoiding long-term complications. As can be seen from the case study, this man's priority was to avoid hypoglycaemia. It is of course easier to accept his decision once the health care team understand what is behind his 'informed choice'. However members of the health care team might still want to find a way of 'fixing things' for this patient. It is in the nature of nursing and medicine to desire to improve our patients' health. In diabetes care it is vital to ensure that the patient's choice is an informed one and to accept that the only person with control over a patient's life is that patient.

How can we develop the ability to facilitate patient self-responsibility? First by taking a person-centred approach and secondly by integrating counselling skills into our patient consultations.

A PERSON-CENTRED APPROACH

Person-centredness is a philosophy of counselling and of education founded by the American psychologist Carl Rogers. His basic premise was that the individual, usually termed client, '... is basically a trustworthy organism, capable of evaluating the outer and inner situation, understanding him or herself in its context, making constructive choices as to the next steps, and acting on those choices' (Rogers 1978).

His philosophy is that the person, not the problem, is the focus in counselling. Some beliefs of a person-centred practitioner are that:

- Human nature is essentially constructive.
- People do their best to grow and to preserve themselves given their internal and external circumstances.
- It is important to reject the pursuit of authority or control over others and seek to share power (Mearns & Thorne 1988).

Self-responsibility and personal growth can be assisted in a relationship where the person-centred practitioner exhibits three core conditions or qualities as being therapeutic in themselves. The core conditions are:

- genuineness
- empathy
- acceptance.

These are communicated to the client through the use of counselling skills.

Genuineness

This quality is also known as realness or congruence. Being genuine is a matter of being oneself with the client. Genuineness or congruence exists where the counsellor responds as he or she feels with regard to the person being counselled. There is no falseness in the relationship. Role playing or attempts to adopt a caring attitude when it is not felt by the counsellor would also prevent the counsellor from being genuine.

Empathy

To have empathy means to comprehend truly and identify with another person's experience. True empathy comes from exploring with the client the exact nature of his/her experience (Nichols 1993). With skilful listening it is sometimes possible to develop a strong sense of what it might be like to be that person. Having the ability to enter the world of the client is called empathy. It is *not* relating the client's experience to your own similar experience.

Acceptance

This is also known as being non-judgemental or having unconditional positive regard. The accepting counsellor values and has a deep regard for the humanity of the client. This regard goes beyond, and is unaffected by, the behaviours of the client which may otherwise be seen as negative, destructive or self-defeating. This attitude of the counsellor is a consistent one, not only with the same client, but with different clients (Mearns & Thorne 1988).

WHAT IS COUNSELLING?

In some ways it is easier to say what counselling is not. Counselling is not about giving advice. Counselling is not about solving people's emotional problems and counselling is not about stopping people's distress.

The following definition of counselling will help to clarify the philosophy of what counselling is:

> Counselling is a process through which one person helps another by *purposeful conversation* in an *understanding atmosphere*. It aims to establish a

helping relationship, in which the one counselled can *express his thoughts and feelings* in such a way as to *clarify* his own situation, come to terms with some new experience, and see his difficulty more objectively and so face his problems with less anxiety and tension. Its basic purpose is to assist the individual to make his own decision from the choices available to him (Royal College of Nursing 1978).

Let's analyse the definition in a bit more detail.

The purposeful conversation

Counselling is often regarded as a 'chat' about psycho-social issues. What can often happen in this situation is that the 'chat' or 'counselling' consists of a number of closed questions which the nurse might think are relevant to the patient's well-being but do not allow the patient to expand, or express new material. Counselling is a precise way of communicating with someone. There are many counselling skills which can be used to facilitate a person-centred approach.

An understanding atmosphere

In counselling it is important to set aside a dedicated time for that patient. It helps the patient to know how much time he/she has as patients often feel pressurised by the thought of others waiting to be seen. Likewise the time spent should be uninterrupted. Surroundings should be comfortable, not too hot or too cold, free from noise and seats placed in such a way that allows a sense of easy communication. The person-centred practitioner is paramount in creating an understanding atmosphere.

Clarification and expression of thoughts and feelings

Often people are muddled about problems that they are experiencing and counselling skills are used to help them make more sense of what is happening to them. This is not only from an emotional standpoint but also to clarify the facts of a problem more clearly. This is further developed in the section on Counselling Skills.

The helping relationship

It is in the nature of nursing to do for patients that which they cannot do for themselves. When with a distressed patient it is only natural that nurses might want to make things better for them. One way of doing this might be to persuade a patient to adopt a solution that the nurse considers best for him. There are two reasons why this rarely works. The first reason is that no matter how much the patient has told you about the problem, some of the facts, because of the nature of distress, will either be distorted or left out. The second reason is that usually the patient will instinctively know if a solution is the right one or not. If 'prescribed' a treatment for the problem which is the wrong treatment, the patient will not follow it.

> *Nurse*: I think the best thing you could do is talk to your husband about your worries and I'm sure you will find that he will be very understanding.
> *Patient* (thinking to herself): I couldn't possibly discuss it. He would go mad, (and then out loud): Yes Nurse, if you think that is the best thing to do.

Here is an alternative dialogue where the nurse suggests a possible solution but in such a way that allows the patient to accept or reject it.

> *Nurse*: What would happen if you talked to your husband about your worries?
> *Patient*: Oh no Nurse, he wouldn't be at all understanding. He would go mad if he knew about my worries.

The helping relationship is a partnership between nurse and patient where the patient uses his/her own power and expertise facilitated by the nurse, and makes his/her own decisions.

COUNSELLING SKILLS

Open invitation to talk

In helping the patient to talk about his difficulties, it is important to structure the questions in such a way that the patient does not respond with a 'yes' or a 'no'. For example, 'What would you like to talk about today?' or 'How have things been since we last met?' Questions that begin with words such as What, How, Could you, Can you, are called open questions. It allows the patient to start where he wants to start. A closed question will come from the frame of reference of the questioner. Closed questions are often looking for very specific information, for example, 'How old are you?', 'Are you married?', 'What is your job?' (Egan 1986).

Verbal following

Verbal following means responding to whatever the client has been saying at that time or earlier on in the session. The counsellor does not need to introduce new topics; the client will set his/her own agenda and the counsellor follows. The counsellor should feel no pressure to 'keep the conversation going'. If the client is silent then the counsellor can be silent too or the silence can be acknowledged, e.g. 'Sometimes it can be difficult to know what to say.'

Paraphrasing

Paraphrasing is where the counsellor repeats to the client what has been said, but in the counsellor's own words. This has two main functions. The first is that the client will be able to 'hear' with more understanding and insight what he/she has been communicating—especially if the paraphrase is given concisely. Secondly, the client will feel listened to and understood. As with reflecting feeling and summarising, paraphrasing has to be done tentatively so that the client can correct the counsellor if the counsellor has got it wrong. Paraphrasing is not the literal mirroring of what has just been said but crystallises the essence of what has been said.

> *Client*: Everything is in a mess at the moment, my marriage, my job and my diabetes.
> *Counsellor*: It sounds as if you have a lot on your plate at the moment.

Reflecting feelings

In trying to understand what the client experiences emotionally in their situation, feelings can be reflected back to the client. In order to reflect feelings the counsellor must begin with not only recognising and being able to label the feeling correctly but also get the intensity of the feeling right. As a result, the client notices that their feelings are accepted and receiving attention. They can then be stimulated to disclose feelings more and to become more aware of them. Sometimes clients have mixed feelings, which inhibits them from getting a clear picture.

> *Patient*: Diabetes has been the worst thing that has happened to me.
> *Nurse* (*not getting it quite right*): So you've been a bit upset about this?

An alternative and more appropriate response could be:

> *Nurse*: It sounds as if you have been devastated by what has happened?

People show their feelings in different ways, both verbally and non-verbally or a combination of both. Non-verbal communication by a client may be acknowledged by verbal response, for instance:

The patient drums his fingers on the table and appears 'jumpy'.
Nurse: You seem quite agitated about this?

Summarisation

The key purpose of summarisation is to help the patient draw together the thoughts and feelings that have been communicated. When the counsellor uses summarisation the patient's verbal and non-verbal statements will be attended to. This is particularly useful half-way through a consultation if the counsellor feels unclear about what is being communicated. Summarising either part of the way through, or at the end, can clarify thoughts and feelings for both the client and the counsellor. As with other skills, summarising should be done tentatively. Clarifying a problem or difficulty can lead to the client gaining insight and making progress.

> *Counsellor*: I wonder if I could recap the last 10 minutes or so. You started off by saying that everything was 'in a mess' and this included your marriage, your job and your diabetes. You decided to concentrate on talking about your diabetes and we would set aside another time to discuss your work and your marriage. In the last few weeks since you were diagnosed with diabetes you have been finding it difficult to stick to your diet and this is partly because you feel rebellious but also angry, as you believe that having diabetes has affected the way other people think of you, and this includes your husband and your colleagues at work. Is there anything that you would like to change or add?

Whilst the counselling process serves to increase self-esteem and enables the client to think in a more positive way about him or herself, the following exercises can also help.

Positive thinking

It is not unusual to find that a patient or client might think of themselves in very negative terms. For example:

> *Client*: I don't deserve all this attention. I'm sure you have other patients that you would rather see.

This kind of statement might be a symptom of a depression but sometimes it is simply a cultural way of thinking about oneself. One exercise to promote change from negative to positive thinking and to increase self-esteem is to ask the patient to write down five words or phrases that best describe him or herself as a person. They should then decide whether these words or phrases are positive or negative qualities by marking a plus sign or a negative sign next to them (Box 3.2). People who are characteristically negative thinkers and who

---

Box 3.2 Labelling yourself

Make a list of 5 words, phrases and traits that describe you best.

Statements		*Alternative to negative statements*
I am FRIENDLY	+	
I am FAT	–	I am CUDDLY
I am WEAK WILLED	–	I am GENEROUS
I am GOOD HUMOURED	+	
I am BAD TEMPERED AT HOME	–	I am GOOD TEMPERED AT WORK

---

might also have low self-esteem tend to think automatically of their bad points. Ask the patient to cross out the negative statements and replace them with positive ones. It is sometimes quite difficult for people to think good things about themselves and they may need assistance with this. Enabling people to dwell on their strengths helps to raise self-esteem. Encourage the patient to keep his list of positive qualities close at hand and every now and then remind him or herself of them.

Setting personal goals for the future

Setting personal goals helps people to feel positive about the future. Again patients can be asked to write down five personal goals for their future and to number these in order of importance (Box 3.3).

Box 3.3 Setting and discussing personal goals

New windows:

For
- Cut heating bills
- Less worry about rotting window frames
- Add to value of flat
- Last for years

Against
- Cost a lot of money
- No holiday!

Going away on holiday:

For
- I'd have fun
- It would be a much needed break

Against
- I need windows
- I'd worry about the windows for the next 50 weeks!

How these goals might be achieved can be discussed. Goal setting can help to integrate diabetes and associated lifestyle changes into daily life.

Case Study 3.3

One woman wanted to go on a round the world trip. Her doctor suggested that with frequent time changes it would be impossible to manage her diabetes so she had abandoned the idea. She was delighted to hear that her insulin regimen could be adapted to accommodate an erratic eating pattern and this helped lift an underlying anger that her diabetes had prevented her from realising a dream.

Taking stock and setting priorities

Some people have so much going on in their lives that they find themselves overwhelmed with stress. It can help to list all the tasks, expectations and demands made on that person and number them in order of priority. On reflection there may be ways of prioritising expectations, eliminating demands or delegating tasks. Introducing new and beneficial changes can lead to an overall sense of well-being (Box 3.4).

DELIVERY OF PSYCHOLOGICAL CARE—

PROFESSIONAL BARRIERS

'Whose diabetes is it anyway?'

There are a number of fears that nurses have about delivering psychological care. One is the pressure to have a solution for all sorts

---

Box 3.4   Taking stock and setting priorities

Things I Do	*Things I Want to Do*
• full-time work	• play the piano
• husband	• jog
• children	• see friends more often
• Open University degree—POSTPONED	
• secretary of choir—STOPPED	

of major and complicated problems that the patient might present. This way of thinking is not an appropriate way of helping people who are having psychological difficulties. However, switching from the traditional paternalistic way of relating to a patient to a more person-centred way of relating is difficult (Table 3.1). The nurse needs different skills. Those that promote patient self-responsibility and prevent the nurse from 'taking over' are counselling skills.

The patient as the expert?

It is sometimes necessary to hold back the 'expertise' within the health professional to facilitate the expertise of the patient. How is this done? There are many practical aspects of the traditional health professional role that communicate the expertise of the health professional and encourage passivity in the patient. These include the wearing of uniform, sitting across a desk, using jargon and judgemental language such as 'cheating' or 'poor control'. However, it is mainly the nature of the style of communication itself that can block patient expertise. Expertise can be counter-productive to empowerment if it makes the patient feel like a child whilst the health professional acts as if a parent.

The 'can of worms'

Health professionals worry that by acknowledging feelings in their patients they might open up a 'can of worms' or a floodgate of emotions that overwhelm and threaten the health professional and somehow 'damage' the patient. Of course it is possible that a patient might reveal a masked depression or other psychological illness. Here it is important that the patient receives appropriate treatment. However, if the health professional finds himself in an emotionally difficult situation beyond his or her abilities then it is important to refer on. This is especially important if the patient presents a problem which is similar to an unresolved problem within the health professional. The health professional will be aware of local psychological and psychiatric services but most major towns and cities will also have separate counselling services. Most reputable counselling services will have British Association of Counselling approval. Some services will charge a fee but this is often tailored to suit the client concerned.

Another fear of the health care professional is that they may make a patient emotionally unstable. However, if a patient expresses emotion about a problem then that emotion existed beforehand and was not created by the counselling health professional. Active listening is therapeutic to the troubled patient, who can be compared to a pressure cooker full of steam. As the pressure increases, there is the feeling that some kind of explosion or disintegration might occur. Letting some of the steam out in the safety of a counselling situation provides a sense of relief and reduces pressure.

'Do I have the time?'

Psychological care can feel time-consuming especially if emotional problems are detected. The patient with diabetes is not receiving full care if the psycho-social issues are ignored in favour of the purely biological aspects of the disease. The key to comprehensive diabetes care is the integration of counselling skills into everyday routine care and not seeing psychological care as a task to be 'ticked off' once 'applied'.

CONCLUSION

Psychological care of people with diabetes is an essential part of care. All health care professionals involved in diabetes care need to acknowledge and address the influences of psycho-social factors on people's lives and on their self-management, diabetic control and long-term health and quality of life. Community nurses are in a powerful position to view diabetes in a person-centred way rather than a disease-centred way and can enhance the delivery of psychological care by the use of counselling skills.

REFERENCES

Anderson R M 1986 The personal meaning of having diabetes: implications for patient behaviour and education or kicking the bucket theory. Diabetic Medicine 3:85–89
Anderson R M 1995 Patient empowerment and the traditional medical model. Diabetes Care 18:3:412–415
Bandura A 1977 Self efficacy: towards a unifying theory of behaviour change. Psychological Review 84, 191–215
Becker M H 1974 The health belief model and personal health behaviour. Health Education Monographs 2:324–473
Bradley C, Cox T 1978 Stress and health. In: Cox T Stress. Macmillan Education Limited, London
Bradley C, Brown C R, Gamsu D S, Moses J L 1984 Development of scales to measure perceived control of diabetes mellitus and diabetes health beliefs. Diabetic Medicine 1:213–218

Brown F J (in press) Who is in control? Counselling for patient empowerment. Practical Diabetes International

Coles C 1989 Diabetes education: theories of practice. Practical Diabetes 6:199–202

Dunn S M 1987 Psychological issues in diabetes management: blood glucose monitoring and learned helplessness. Practical Diabetes 4:3:108–110

Egan G 1986 The skilled helper. A systematic approach to effective helping. Brooks/Coles Publishing Company, Pacific Grove, California: 31–68

Ewles L, Simnet I 1992 Promoting health: a practical guide. Scutari Press, Middlesex

Feste C 1992 A practical look at patient empowerment. Diabetes Care 15:7:922–925

Funnell M M, Anderson R M, Arnold M S et al 1991 Empowerment: an idea whose time has come in diabetes education. The Diabetes Educator 17:37–41

Holmes T H, Rahe R H 1967 The social readjustment rating scale. Journal of Psychosomatic Research 11:213

Jones A 1992 Gestalt therapy: theory and practice. Nursing Standard 6:38:31–34

Kubler Ross E 1990 On death and dying. Routledge, London

Lancet Editorial 1994 Essence of stress. The Lancet 344:1713–1714

Lawrence R D 1935 A diabetic life (Out of print.)

Lewis K S, Jennings A M, Ward J D, Bradley C 1990 Health belief scales developed specifically for people with tablet-treated Type 2 diabetes. Diabetic Medicine 7:148–155

Mearns D, Thorne B 1988 Person-centred counselling in action. Sage Publications, London: 18, 75

Nichols K A 1993 Psychological care in physical illness, 2nd edn. Chapman and Hall, London

Rogers C 1978 Carl Rogers on personal power. Constable, London: 15

Rogers C 1980 A way of being. Houghton Mifflin Co. Boston

Royal College of Nursing Working Party 1978 Counselling in nursing. Royal College of Nursing, London: 14

Shillitoe R W 1987 Diabetes education: ideas into action. Practical Diabetes 4:3:133–135

Shillitoe R W 1988 Psychology and diabetes. Psychological factors in management and control. Chapman and Hall, London: 119

Stewart W 1992 An A-Z of counselling theory and practice. Chapman and Hall, London: 251–252

Tones K 1991 Health promotion, empowerment and the psychology of control. Journal of the Institute of Health Education 29:1:17–26

Tones K, Tilford S, Robinson Y 1990 Health education: effectiveness and efficiency. Chapman and Hall, London

World Health Organization 1984 Health promotion. A WHO discussion document on the concepts and principles. In Journal of the Institute of Health Education 1985 23:1

The patient with non-insulin-dependent diabetes mellitus

Derek Gordon

4

■ CONTENTS

Non-insulin-dependent diabetes is a disease of insidious onset often discovered during routine screening when the patient may have few if any symptoms. For this reason it is often termed 'mild diabetes', a phrase which should never be used with patients since it implies that their diabetes is not serious and may give a false sense of security. NIDDM patients are at risk of developing diabetic complications and, indeed, may already have well-established complications by the time of diagnosis (see Ch. 2). In particular, such patients are at risk of developing widespread vascular disease which will be the main cause of their premature deaths.

The aims of treatment for NIDDM patients are twofold: control of the blood glucose concentrations and reduction in the risk factors for macrovascular diseases. The management of diabetic control is dealt with in this chapter, while the reduction in macrovascular risk is discussed more fully in Chapter 8.

DIET

Dietary manipulation is fundamental to the management of the patient with NIDDM. The basic tenets of dietary management should therefore be known to the primary health care team so that preliminary advice can be given in the community at the time of diagnosis (Ch. 6). However, few doctors or nurses have adequate training to provide complete dietary advice and all newly diagnosed NIDDM patients should receive additional advice from a trained dietitian.

Well over 50% of all newly diagnosed NIDDM patients in the UK are overweight (BMI 25.0–30.0 kg/m^2) or obese (BMI> 30.0 kg/m^2). The cornerstone to their diet is an individualized low calorie diet (Ch. 6). Eating less reduces energy intake and allows weight reduction. Reduced energy intake in turn results in lower blood glucose concentrations and this may subsequently allow some recovery of pancreatic islet cell function. There is evidence that chronically elevated blood glucose levels are toxic to the islet cells and impair insulin secretion. The exact biochemical mechanisms responsible for this toxic effect of hyperglycaemia are poorly understood (Rossetti et al 1990). Reduction in weight also improves the peripheral insulin resistance which is a feature of NIDDM (Ch. 1). Hence by the reduction in weight, the patient is able to utilise their own insulin production more effectively.

When diet succeeds, the benefits are evident. Blood glucose, lipids and blood pressure fall and life expectancy may be prolonged by 3–4 months for each kg lost during the first year of treatment (Lean et al 1990). If patients can be motivated and are reviewed at frequent intervals by both doctor and dietitian, quite startling results can be achieved. In Belfast, 80% of NIDDM patients who were treated by diet alone and reviewed 3-monthly, remained well controlled after six years (Hadden et al 1986).

The response to diet however is often disappointing. Most diabetic clinics in general practice or hospital lack the resources required to allow such frequent dietary review and patients often lack motivation or find it impossible to alter deeply ingrained eating habits. The UK Prospective Diabetes Study found that only 16% of newly diagnosed NIDDM patients achieved near normal fasting blood glucose concentrations after three months of dieting. Patients with the highest fasting blood glucose levels at the time of diagnosis were least likely to achieve good diabetic control by diet alone (UK Prospective Diabetes Study 7 1990).

Case Study 4.1

A 49-year-old long-distance HGV driver is diagnosed as diabetic when he attends his GP complaining of tiredness. He has no symptoms of polydipsia or polyuria and his weight has remained steady at just over 123 kg (19 stone). He eats very erratically from cheap hot-food stalls or motorway cafeterias. He smokes about 30 cigarettes per day and he never takes any form of exercise. He does not drink alcohol when he is working. However he does admit to enjoying 'a few pints' on a Friday and Saturday night. His GP estimates his weekly alcohol intake at approximately 30 units. He was found to have high blood pressure several years ago and has been taking a thiazide diuretic. His father and two sisters have diabetes and he has an older brother who had a heart attack when he was aged 47 years. Because of this history, his GP checked his random blood glucose and found it to be elevated at 11.8 mmol/l. In order to confirm the diagnosis the GP also arranged for a fasting blood glucose to be measured the following morning. This result was also raised at 8.1 mmol/l.

The finding of two blood glucose concentrations within the diagnostic range confirms that this patient is diabetic and his elevated blood glucose may be the cause of his lethargy. Although his symptoms of diabetes are minimal, his risk of serious illness in the future is by no means small. In addition to his diabetes, his unhealthy lifestyle will further increase the risk of vascular catastrophe in the future unless he makes major alterations to the way he lives.

His case history is fairly typical of the NIDDM patient. There is a strong family history of NIDDM and he has the associated risk factor of being overweight. With his lifestyle and family history of cardiac disease he is also at high risk of cardiovascular problems. Hence his initial management would be by diet and encouragement to make the appropriate lifestyle changes.

The patient is hypertensive and should be advised to restrict his intake of salt to around 3 g/24 h. This can usually be achieved by limiting the use of salt to cooking and not adding salt at the table. The patient should be aware that many proprietary foods are high in salt content. With the additional family history of ischaemic heart disease, our patient should be screened for hyperlipidaemia and given additional dietary advice if required. Further assistance should be given to help him to stop smoking and he should be encouraged to start regular exercise.

A change to his anti-hypertensive therapy would also be advised since this may be contributing to his glucose intolerance. Thiazide diuretics increase the resistance of the tissues of the body to the action of insulin. This unwanted side-effect will therefore worsen the blood glucose control. It should be remembered that patients with NIDDM are usually middle-aged or elderly and may be suffering from other medical conditions at the time of diagnosis. They may be taking other medications which interfere with their diabetes and a careful review of their medication at the time of diagnosis is mandatory. This subject will be dealt with more fully below.

Case Study 4.2

A 62-year-old female who has had NIDDM for 8 years has maintained good metabolic control by dietary measures until recently. Over the past 2 months her urine testing results have become persistently positive for glucose and she has developed symptoms of polydipsia and polyuria. She has never been significantly overweight (BMI 23.0 kg/m^2) and she has lost a few kg recently. She denies any change in her dietary compliance. A blood glucose estimation at the clinic is 18.9 mmol/l and a glycosylated haemoglobin result confirms a recent deterioration in control.

Before starting therapy with an oral hypoglycaemic agent further dietary assessment should be undertaken to ensure compliance and motivation. A patient who is poorly compliant with diet is unlikely to achieve satisfactory metabolic control with tablets. Because this particular patient is not obese, a sulphonylurea would be the class of hypoglycaemic agent to choose.

THE SULPHONYLUREAS

The sulphonylureas have been used to treat NIDDM for more than 30 years. Despite this, our knowledge of their mode of action is limited. The major action of sulphonylureas is to lower blood glucose concentrations by stimulating the beta cells of the pancreas to secrete insulin. Therefore the effect of sulphonylureas is limited to patients with preserved pancreatic cell function. (A feature of NIDDM is the gradual loss of islet cell function—see Ch. 1). The pancreas can only be squeezed to produce more insulin if there is insulin there to be squeezed!

Sulphonylureas are therefore likely to be most effective early in the course of NIDDM. However, they are often not used until diet has failed completely—by which time they may be relatively ineffective in some patients. Therefore a 3-month trial of diet should be carried out and if blood glucose levels are not adequately controlled by that time a sulphonylurea should be introduced. The sulphonylureas also have minor 'extra-pancreatic' effects on glucose metabolism but these effects are probably of little clinical significance.

It is generally recommended that sulphonylureas are ingested about 30 minutes before meals as this will stimulate insulin production to coincide with the time of eating. This in turn has been shown to reduce the post-prandial rise in blood glucose (Melander et al 1989). Most drugs of this group are given twice daily when used at higher doses. The maximum therapeutic effect of most sulphonylureas is achieved at relatively low doses. This is presumably because the cell receptors for the drug become saturated at low doses and further increases in drug dose have no additional effects. A patient who shows poor glycaemic control on a dose of gliclazide 160 mg daily, glibenclamide or glipizide 10 mg daily is unlikely to respond to higher doses and a decision to start insulin therapy should not be delayed unnecessarily.

There is little evidence to support that one compound is more effective than another and little to be gained from changing from one sulphonylurea to another (Cohen & Harris 1987; Groop 1992; Sonksen et al 1981).

When initiating sulphonylurea treatment in the elderly, care should be taken to start with the smallest possible dose, e.g. gliclazide 40 mg, glipizide 2.5 mg, etc. Patients should be advised to eat regular meals and they should also be told about the signs and symptoms of hypo-glycaemia so that they can recognise them and take appropriate action. If a patient forgets to take a morning dose then the correct advice is to take the tablet just prior to the next meal and not to take it on an empty stomach when food is not imminent.

The most important side-effect with this group of compounds is the development of serious and prolonged hypoglycaemia. For this reason, any patient who becomes hypoglycaemic due to a sulphonylurea should be admitted to hospital for at least 24 hours for observation and management. The elderly are most at risk, probably because of coexisting vascular disease of the brain and heart. Almost all severe cases of prolonged hypoglycaemia have involved patients over the age of 70 years (Ferner & Neil 1988; Jennings et al 1979). Of those admitted to hospital with sulphonylurea-induced hypoglycaemia, 10% will die and 3% will be left with permanent brain damage. The incidence of serious hypoglycaemic episodes is higher with the longer acting preparations, chlorpropamide and glibenclamide, and these drugs should be avoided in the elderly (Seltzer 1979).

Alcohol consumption, poor food intake, renal impairment, and drugs which potentiate sulphonylureas' actions may contribute to hypoglycaemic problems. Drugs interfering with the action of sulphonylureas are listed in Table 4.1.

The other common side-effect of sulphonylureas is unwanted weight gain and for this reason they are not the drugs of first choice in the obese diabetic. Table 4.2 lists the most commonly used sulphonylureas along with their usual daily doses and their duration of action.

THE BIGUANIDES

Case Study 4.3

A 72-year-old female patient with NIDDM has been overweight almost all of her life. She is troubled by arthritis of her hips and knees and her mobility has progressively deteriorated over recent years. Accordingly, her weight has been gradually rising and she now finds herself weighing 104 kg (16 stone—BMI 32 kg/m^2). Her diabetes was diagnosed when she presented with significant symptoms of hyperglycaemia. Despite attempts to diet over a 3-month period, she has been unable to lose weight and her blood glucose results remain significantly elevated.

This obese patient may respond to biguanide therapy.

The history of this class of diabetic medication can be traced back to medieval times when *Galega officinalis* (goat's rue or French lilac) was used as a traditional remedy for diabetes in southern and

Table 4.1 Drugs influencing diabetic control

Hypoglycaemic effects	Hyperglycaemic effects	Interactions with sulphonylureas
Alcohol	Corticosteroids	Sulphonamides #
MAOI	Thiazide and loop diuretics	Trimethoprim#
Fibrates	Chlorpromazine	Chloramphenicol#
Miconazole	Chronic alcohol	Ciprofloxin#.
Salicylates	Oral contraceptives	
Cimetidine, ranitidine	Anabolic steroids	Rifampicin*

enhance action of sulphonylureas
* antagonise action of sulphonylureas

eastern Europe. This plant was subsequently shown to be rich in guanidine and in 1918 guanidine was shown to have mild hypoglycaemic effects. However guanidine was too toxic for clinical use and it was not until the 1950s that biguanide derivatives were introduced into clinical practice. Two biguanides, phenformin and metformin, were extensively used. Phenformin was later shown to have been associated with the development of lactic acidosis, a potentially fatal side-effect in some patients, and this led to the withdrawal of this compound from clinical used in many countries including the UK. Metformin is therefore the only biguanide available for the treatment of diabetes in this country.

Table 4.2 The more commonly used sulphonylureas

Drug	Effect duration (Hours)	Daily dose (mg)
Tolbutamide	6–10	500–3000
Gliclazide	10–15	40–320
Glipizide	14–16	2.5–20
Glibenclamide	20–24	2.5–20
Chlorpropamide	24–72	100–500

Metformin

Metformin, in contrast to sulphonylureas, does not cause clinical hypoglycaemia. This drug lowers blood glucose concentrations by several mechanisms. The glucose-lowering effect occurs without stimulation of insulin secretion and results mainly from enhanced insulin action on the peripheral tissues, particularly muscle. In addition, metformin reduces the absorption of glucose from the intestine and inhibits the production of glucose by the liver. It may also have direct or indirect effects reducing appetite (Bailey 1992).

Metformin is likely to reduce blood glucose concentrations by 2–3 mmol/l when prescribed for patients who have failed on diet. About 30% of patients so treated will achieve good diabetic control. However, a further 5–10% of patients will fail on treatment each year due to poor dietary or drug compliance.

Metformin is available as 500 and 850 mg tablets. The drug should be taken with meals and the dose increased gradually in order to lessen side-effects. A typical starting dose would be 850 mg once daily or 500 mg twice daily. The maximum recommended daily dose is 3 g (1 g with each meal), although this dosage is usually poorly tolerated by most patients.

The most common side-effects of metformin are gastrointestinal in origin. About 20% of patients experience diarrhoea, flatulence or abdominal pain, while others may complain of metallic taste, nausea or anorexia. A reduction in appetite may be desirable in the overweight patient but for the sake of compliance must be seriously considered. These disturbances are generally transient and can be minimized by starting treatment at low dosage and taking the drug along with food.

Metformin can cause the blood lactate levels to rise. This is usually slight and of no clinical significance. However, serious lactic acidosis can occur if metformin is prescribed for unsuitable patients. Metformin is normally excreted through the kidneys and is contraindicated in patients with renal impairment (e.g. serum creatinine > 120 µmol/l) since this can result in accumulation of the drug in the body, enhancing its effect on lactic acid production. Liver disease is also a contraindication, since adequate hepatic function is required to metabolize the increased lactic acid. Patients with cardiac failure perfuse their tissues poorly and the resulting tissue hypoxia causes lactic acid production. It is therefore unwise to prescribe metformin for such patients.

Because of the fear of lactic acidosis, many European countries restrict the use of metformin to patients under the age of 65 or 70 years. This has been endorsed by the European NIDDM Policy Group, which has stated that metformin should not be prescribed for patients over 65 years of age (Alberti & Gries 1988). However, metformin can be safely prescribed in the elderly without risk of lactic acidosis if strict adherence to the prescribing guidelines is practised: that is, it should not be used in patients with renal or hepatic dysfunction or patients with cardiac or respiratory failure (Chalmers et al 1992).

COMBINATION THERAPY—SULPHONYLUREA PLUS METFORMIN

If monotherapy with either a sulphonylurea or metformin fails to control blood glucose it is logical to consider combination therapy. The sulphonylurea stimulates insulin secretion and metformin enhances the action of insulin upon the peripheral cells. Combination therapy should therefore be more effective than either drug alone. An early study confirmed that up to 50% of patients not controlled by high sulphonylurea dose improved substantially when metformin was added (Clarke & Duncan 1979). However, in clinical practice, the thin patient failing on sulphonylureas is probably in need of insulin and the benefit of combination therapy may be short-lived. Similarly, the obese patient failing on metformin is probably poorly compliant with diet, and combination therapy, while still worthwhile trying, may simply cause further weight gain.

OTHER DRUGS AVAILABLE FOR NIDDM

There are other preparations available which may help in the management of NIDDM. These agents have no effect on insulin production nor on glucose metabolism but serve to demonstrate the complex nature of NIDDM!

The alpha-glucosidase inhibitors

Acerbose is the only drug of this class presently available in the UK, although it is likely that newer alpha-glucosidase inhibitors will become available in the near future. Alpha-glucosidases are enzymes which line the gut wall and are required for the absorption of various carbohydrates. Inhibition of these enzymes by acerbose results in delayed absorption of carbohydrate. Several studies have shown that acerbose can reduce post-prandial hyperglycaemia when used alone or in combination with a sulphonylurea (Hotta et al 1993, Sachse 1988). Acerbose is poorly tolerated with a high incidence of gastrointestinal side-effects, mainly flatulence and abdominal distension. These side-effects can be reduced by starting treatment at a low dosage: 50 mg once daily and gradually building up the dose to 50 mg three times daily over a period of a week or two. The tablets should be taken with food and chewed slowly. Patients should be advised about side-effects when the drug is started and encouraged to persevere since tolerance often develops over a period of about a month. The maximum dose is 100 mg three times daily. Acerbose may be of particular value in patients for whom metformin is contraindicated.

Appetite suppressants

Appetite suppressants have often been frowned upon by the medical profession. There is a widely held belief that while they may reduce weight initially, they do not alter the obese patient's long-term eating habits and any benefits obtained are temporary. However, the management of the overweight NIDDM patient who has not responded to diet or metformin is a challenge to all concerned. The addition of sulphonylurea or insulin therapy may result in further substantial weight gain without improvement in metabolic control. The use of appetite suppression in these patients should therefore be considered.

Dexfenfluramine has been shown to cause a significant reduction in weight over a period of 3 months when used on obese NIDDM patients (Willey et al 1992). In addition NIDDM patients treated with dexfenfluramine achieved significant improvements in glycaemic control and this improvement appeared to be independent of the amount of weight loss (Scheen et al 1991). This drug may therefore have an additional and more specific action influencing diabetic control. Dexfenfluramine is licensed only for a 3-month course in any one year and its potential for sustained therapeutic benefit in NIDDM patients may therefore be limited.

Fluoxetine is an antidepressant with similar pharmacology to dexfenfluramine. This drug is not limited to 3-month courses and more prolonged trials of its efficacy in causing weight reduction have been possible. Fluoxetine can cause significant weight reduction over a period of 12 months in obese NIDDM patients. However improved glycaemic control was maintained for only 6 months (O'Kane et al 1994). The place for appetite suppressants in the management of obese NIDDM patients therefore remains controversial, and further, more prolonged trials are required in order to determine their position.

Guar gum

Preparations of guar gum were in vogue several years ago for the treatment of NIDDM. Guar gum is a natural soluble fibre which, after ingestion, forms a viscous gel which slows gastric emptying and retards carbohydrate absorption from the intestine. When taken before meals it can reduce post-prandial glucose peaks. However, its hypoglycaemic action is weak. Its side-effects of flatulence, abdominal bloating and diarrhoea made it unpopular and it is little used now.

INSULIN THERAPY

Case Study 4.4

A 68-year-old woman has had NIDDM for 15 years. She was treated initially by diet alone and subsequently with a sulphonylurea. Four years ago metformin was added to her drug regimen because her diabetic control deteriorated. Although this improved her urine testing results, they remained mainly at 1%. She is presently taking gliclazide 160 mg twice daily and metformin 1 g twice daily. She is unable to tolerate a higher dose of metformin because of symptoms of diarrhoea and abdominal pain. She has never been overweight, and recently her weight has gradually been falling. She has lost 6 kg in weight over the past year. She is symptomatic with polydipsia and nocturia. The need for insulin therapy has been discussed with her on several occasions but she is reluctant to consider this option.

The thin NIDDM patient who is symptomatic and losing weight has reached the point where the pancreatic beta cells have failed and the patient is insulin-deficient. Insulin therapy will correct the insulin deficiency and reduce blood glucose levels. This in turn will reduce the toxic effects of chronically high glucose levels and insulin resistance, and endogenous insulin secretion may improve.

Many patients have a deep-seated fear of self-injection and are understandably reluctant to consider insulin treatment. It can be explained that insulin will be given for a trial period and can subsequently be withdrawn if the patient so wishes. This often acts to reassure the patient who feels that the introduction of insulin treatment is a 'life sentence'. Most patients requiring insulin therapy are tired and lethargic, although they may not appreciate the significance of these symptoms, attributing them to old age. It is important to point out to the doubting patient that insulin therapy may give them a new lease of life. Most patients started on insulin treatment feel so much better; their symptoms of polydipsia and polyuria recede, they regain lost weight, and they generally feel more energetic. Most patients 'never look back' after starting insulin therapy and do not contemplate reverting to oral therapy.

Case Study 4.5

This patient is also a 68-year-old woman who has been diabetic for 5 years. She weighs 117 kg (18 stone—BMI> 30) and has been unable to lose weight on diet or metformin treatment. Gliclazide was introduced about 1 year ago. This improved metabolic control initially but resulted in weight gain of nearly 6.5 kg (1 stone) over a 6-month period. The dose of gliclazide has been increased to maximum without further benefit and the patient's blood glucose levels at the clinic are usually greater than 17 mmol/l. Our patient is troubled by recurrent carbuncles and persistent vaginal thrush.

This patient is markedly obese and likely to be insulin resistant. The pancreatic cells may still be functioning well and producing normal or even increased amounts of insulin. Will such a patient benefit from insulin therapy? Attempts to achieve control of blood glucose may result in massive doses of insulin being prescribed. This in turn can result in rapid weight gain. In this particular case the patient is plagued by recurrent skin infections which have resulted from her poor metabolic control. Weight gain may be the price she has to pay in order to reduce the discomfort of repeated infections. Every effort should be made to encourage weight loss by dieting and exercise, and the use of an appetite suppressant may be justified.

In other cases the patient may be so discouraged by weight gain, which may be unsightly and causes reduced mobility, that he or she may opt for a return to oral agents. The goal of tight metabolic control is rarely achieved in such patients and insulin therapy has little to offer.

Most general practices will refer patients requiring insulin therapy to the local hospital diabetic clinic. The principles of insulin therapy in NIDDM will be briefly described here and the reader is referred to Chapter 5 where the subject is dealt with in greater depth. Once-daily long-acting or intermediate-acting insulin (e.g. lente or isophane) can be tried, particularly in the elderly patient who may require community nursing assistance with injections. However, for the majority of patients the aim is to achieve optimum metabolic control and such regimens are rarely adequate (Peacock & Tattersall 1984). If once-daily isophane insulin is used, there is some evidence that better overall control of the diabetes can be achieved if the insulin is given at bedtime rather than before breakfast (Seigler et al 1992). In clinical practice however insulin is rarely prescribed in this manner possibly because of fear that insulin given before bed might cause nocturnal hypoglycaemia. Tight glycaemic control can be achieved using twice-daily isophane and soluble insulin injections. It should always be remembered that patients with NIDDM tend to be resistant to the action of insulin and a large daily insulin dosage may be necessary in order to overcome this insulin resistance (Genuth 1990; Henry et al 1993).

Insulin plus sulphonylureas

In patients capable of partial response to sulphonylureas, the combination of sulphonylurea plus insulin might achieve better glycaemic control. Since the sulphonylureas stimulate endogenous insulin secretion, lower insulin doses might be expected to be effective. In practice, the effects of combined insulin-sulphonylurea therapy on glycaemic control are modest (Pugh et al 1992). The advantage of reduced insulin dose is offset by the added complexity of patients requiring to take both oral medication and insulin. Such combined regimens are rarely used in clinical practice.

Insulin plus metformin

For the obese patient poorly controlled on insulin therapy the introduction of metformin might seem logical. Metformin improves the action of insulin on peripheral tissues and one would expect it to reduce the requirement for high doses of insulin in this type of patient. The addition of metformin to insulin therapy might also be expected to reduce or prevent the inevitable weight gain which occurs in the obese NIDDM patient following the introduction of insulin therapy. It is perhaps surprising therefore that very little has been written on this subject and only one research paper has been published showing the results of such combination treatment in elderly, obese, insulin-treated diabetic patients who had previously failed on oral therapy (Giugliano et al 1993). This group showed that the addition of metformin to insulin treatment resulted in improved diabetic control with smaller doses of insulin. The effect of combination therapy on their patients' weights was however not reported. Clearly more studies are required to determine the long-term benefits of such a regimen.

DRUGS OF THE FUTURE

Currently available oral hypoglycaemic agents are not completely successful in achieving close metabolic control in NIDDM. New medications are required, particularly for the patients who respond poorly to diet, drugs and insulin treatment. Obesity is perhaps the major obstacle to effective treatment, and novel anti-obesity drugs are being investigated. Some of these preparations stimulate energy expenditure. Others inhibit the appetite centre of the brain. New alpha-glucosidase inhibitors may become available. Drugs which stimulate the release of insulin and others which sensitise the tissues to the action of insulin are being investigated. Finally drugs which interfere with the metabolism of glucose by inhibiting enzymes required for glucose production are also under investigation (Bressler & Johnson 1992).

MEDICATIONS ALTERING GLUCOSE TOLERANCE AND DRUG INTERACTIONS

The patient with NIDDM will be middle-aged or elderly and may have other medical conditions which are being treated simultaneously. As stated elsewhere, NIDDM patients often have hypertension, hyperlipidaemia and vascular disease. Such patients may commonly be taking medications which interfere with their diabetes (Table 4.1).

Hyperglycaemic effects

Thiazide diuretics such as bendrofluazide are known to increase blood glucose levels by causing increased resistance to the action of insulin on peripheral tissues. Remember that thiazide diuretics are often included in 'combination pills' such as Tenoretic, Capozide, etc.

The loop diuretics frusemide and bumetanide also have mild effects on glucose tolerance.

The beta-blockers are another group of drugs frequently used for the treatment of hypertension and angina and therefore commonly prescribed for diabetic patients. These drugs also impair glucose tolerance and may worsen diabetic control.

Blood glucose levels can be increased by oestrogen-containing preparations or drugs with oestrogen-like actions. The oral contraceptives are not often used in this age-group. However, hormone replacement therapy is used in this population and must be introduced with care in the older female with NIDDM lest diabetic control is allowed to deteriorate. The anti-oestrogen tamoxifen does have oestrogenic effects also, and can worsen glucose tolerance. This medication is commonly used in the older patient with breast malignancy.

Corticosteroids antagonise the action of insulin and therefore medications such as prednisolone used for the treatment of asthma or for immunosuppression will result in raising blood glucose concentrations. Anabolic steriods are used in some patients with malignancy and are also used illegally for body building. They too will cause blood glucose levels to rise.

Adrenaline is another hormone which can counter the action of insulin and it is important to remember that adrenaline or adrenaline-like compounds (phenylpropanolamine and ephedrine) are frequently found in decongestants and cold remedies.

Hypoglycaemic effects

Other drugs can have hypoglycaemic effects. Aspirin and other non-steroidal anti-inflammatory agents have a mild blood glucose lowering effect. Similarly, alcohol can cause hypoglycaemia particularly if a patient is taking insulin or on sulphonylurea treatment. Alcohol acts on the liver and reduces the ability of the liver to produce glucose. Hence alcohol will enhance the hypoglycaemic effects of insulin or oral hypoglycaemic agents.

Drugs interfering with the action of sulphonylureas

Drugs which bind to proteins in the blood can displace the sulphony-lureas from their binding sites and release more active drug into the circulation thus causing hypoglycaemia. The sulphonamide antibiotics and trimethoprim are examples of drugs which compete with the sulphonylureas from their protein binding sites. Other antibiotics such as chloramphenicol and the 4-quinolones can also enhance the hypoglycaemic action of the sulphonylureas. Rifampicin on the other hand is an antibiotic which accelerates the metabolism of the sulphonylureas and therefore reduces their therapeutic effect. A list of medications which can alter the hypoglycaemic effects of the sulphonylureas is also given in Table 4.1, page 67.

UK PROSPECTIVE DIABETES STUDY

Little is known about the long-term benefits of drug or insulin therapy in NIDDM. In order to determine whether improved diabetic control influences the development of diabetic complications, the UK Prospective Diabetes Study (UKPDS) was started in 1977 and since then, over 6000 patients have been recruited throughout Great Britain. The study also aims to identify the most effective treatment regimen for NIDDM (UKPDS 1991).

This study has recently compared the effect of diet alone with various treatments in both obese and non-obese NIDDM patients over the first three years following diagnosis (UKPDS Group 1995). Non-obese patients were treated by either diet alone or diet with chlorpropamide, or glibenclamide or once-daily insulin injections. Obese patients received dietary advice with or without the addition of chlorpropamide or glibenclamide or insulin or metformin. The study aimed to maintain fasting blood glucose concentrations below 7.8 mmol/l.

Over the first 3 years only 23% of those allocated to diet achieved the target for fasting blood glucose concentrations. By contrast over half the patients on drug therapy achieved fasting blood glucose levels below 7.8 mmol/l and significantly lower glycated haemoglobin levels were obtained by patients receiving drugs. In the non-obese patients there was very little to choose between the different drug regimens. Chlorpropamide may have been slightly more effective than glibenclamide, causing less minor hypoglycaemic incidents and less weight gain. However, all drug treatments in this group caused weight increase when compared to diet alone.

The obese group perhaps not unexpectedly proved less responsive to all treatments. The sulphonylureas and insulin caused further weight gain. Metformin however did not result in excessive weight gain compared to diet alone.

The first 3 years' data from this mammoth study have regrettably been unable to identify the most effective treatment for NIDDM patients and more prolonged follow-up will be necessary before it will be possible to establish whether any particular therapy is better than any other for reducing the risk of long-term complications.

CONCLUSION

A treatment algorithm for NIDDM is shown in Figure 4.1. Dietary management is fundamental to the care of all patients with NIDDM. All patients should benefit from the advice of a qualified dietitian at the time of diagnosis. Only when diet has failed to produce adequate control should drug therapy be considered. Sulphonylureas are the drugs of first choice for non-obese patients. The dosage should be increased as necessary. Remember however that there is little additional hypoglycaemic effect with maximum doses, and other therapies should be considered. The addition of metformin is advantageous for some patients. However, if the patient is thin and losing weight he or she probably requires insulin therapy and there is nothing to be gained by unnecessary delay in instituting this treatment.

For the obese patient, metformin is the drug of choice but health care staff should beware of other medical problems which may contraindicate its use. Liver function and serum creatinine should be regularly monitored while patients are taking metformin. Sulphonylureas can be added to the treatment regimen if diet and metformin are unsuccessful. Sulphonylureas may cause further weight gain with subsequent deterioration in glycaemic control. Under these circumstances a trial of insulin therapy is justified. However, this may simply cause more weight gain without improvement in diabetic control. If this occurs, despite further encouragement to diet, it may be necessary to compromise and accept that tight metabolic control will not be achieved.

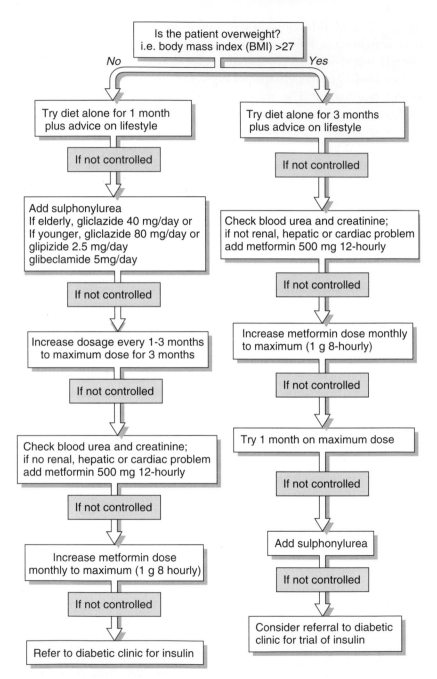

Fig. 4.1 The management of NIDDM.

REFERENCES

Alberti K G M M, Gries F A 1988 Management of non-insulin-dependent diabetes mellitus in Europe: a consensus view. Diabetic Medicine 5:275–281

Bailey C J 1992 Biguanides and NIDDM. Diabetes Care 15:755–772

Bressler R, Johnson D 1992 New pharmacological approaches to therapy of NIDDM. Diabetes Care 6:792–804

Cohen K L, Harris S 1987 Efficacy of glyburide in diabetics poorly controlled on first-generation oral hypoglycemics. Diabetes Care 10:555–557

Chalmers J, Brown I R F, McBain A M, Campbell I W 1992 Metformin: is its use contraindicated in the elderly? Practical Diabetes 9:51–53

Clarke B F, Duncan L J P 1979 Biguanide treatment in the management of insulin dependent (maturity-onset) diabetes; clinical experience with metformin. Research and Clinical Forums 1:53–63

Ferner R E, Neil H A W 1988 Sulphonylureas and hypoglycaemia (editorial). British Medical Journal 296:949–950

Genuth S 1990 Insulin use in NIDDM. Diabetes Care 13:1240–1264

Groop L C 1992 Sulphonylureas in NIDDM. Diabetes Care 15:737–754

Giugliano D, Quatraro A, Consoli G et al 1993 Metformin for obese, insulin-treated diabetic patients: improvement in glycaemic control and reduction of metabolic risk factors. European Journal of Clinical Pharmacology 44:107–112

Hadden D R, Blair A L T, Wilson E A et al 1986 Natural history of diabetes presenting age 40–69 years: a prospective study of the influence of intensive dietary therapy. Quarterly Journal of Medicine 59:574–598

Henry R R, Gumbiner B, Ditzler T, Wallace P et al 1993 Intensive conventional insulin therapy for type II diabetes. Diabetes Care 16:21–31

Hotta N, Kakuta H, Sano T, Matsumae H, Yamada H, Kitazawa S, Sakamoto N 1993 Long-term effect of acerbose on glycaemic control in non-insulin-dependent diabetes mellitus: a placebo controlled double-blind study. Diabetic Medicine 10:134–138

Jennings A M, Wilson R M, Ward J D 1989 Symptomatic hypoglycemia in NIDDM patients treated with oral hypoglycemic agents. Diabetes Care 12:203–205

Lean M E J, Powrie J K, Anderson A S, Garthwaite P H 1990 Obesity, weight loss and prognosis in Type 2 diabetes. Diabetic Medicine 7:228–233

Melander A, Bitzen P-O, Faber O, Groop L 1989 Sulphonylurea antidiabetic drugs: An update of their clinical pharmacology and rational therapeutic use. Drugs 37:58–72

O'Kane M, Wiles P G, Wales J K 1994 Fluoxetine in the treatment of obese type 2 diabetic patients. Diabetic Medicine 11:105–110

Peacock I, Tattersall R B 1984 The difficult choice of treatment for poorly controlled maturity onset diabetes: tablets or insulin? British Medical Journal 288: 1956–1959

Pugh J A, Wagner M L, Sawyer J, Ramirez G, Tuley M, Friedberg S J 1992 Combination sulfonylurea and insulin therapy useful in NIDDM patients? Diabetes care 15:953–959

Rossetti L, Giaccari A, DeFronzo R A 1990 Glucose toxicity. Diabetes Care 13:610–630

Sachse G 1988 Acerbose for the treatment of diabetes mellitus. Acerbose in non-insulin dependent diabetes – long-term studies in combination with oral agents. In: Creutzfeld W (ed) 2nd International symposium on acerbose, Berlin, 12–14 November 1987. Springer-Verlag, Heidelberg: 92–101

Scheen A J, Paolisso G, Salvatore T, Lefebvre P J 1991 Improvement of insulin-induced glucose disposal in obese patients with NIDDM after 1-week treatment with d-fenfluramine. Diabetes Care 14:325–332

Seigler D E, Olsson G M, Skyler J S 1992 Morning versus bedtime isophane insulin in type 2 (non-insulin dependent) diabetes mellitus. Diabetic Medicine 9:826–833

Seltzer H S 1979 Severe drug-induced hypoglycemia: a review. Comprehensive
    Therapy 5:21–29
Sonksen P H, Lowry C, Perkins J R, West T E T 1981 Hormonal and metabolic effects
    of chlorpropamine, glibenclamide and placebo in a crossover study in diabetics not
    controlled by diet alone. Diabetologia 20:22–30
UK Prospective Diabetes Study 7 1990 Response of fasting plasma glucose to diet
    therapy in newly presenting type II diabetic patients. Metabolism 39:905–912
UK Prospective Diabetes Study 8 1991 Study design, progress and performance.
    Diabetologia 34:877–890
UK Prospective Diabetes Study 13 1995 Relative efficacy of randomly allocated diet,
    sulphonylurea, insulin, or metformin in patients with newly diagnosed non-insulin
    dependent diabetes followed for three years. British Medical Journal 310:83–88
Willey K A, Molyneaux L M, Overland J E, Yue D K 1992 The effects of
    dexfenfluramine on blood glucose control in patients with type 2 diabetes. Diabetic
    Medicine 9:341–343

The patient with insulin-dependent diabetes mellitus

Derek Gordon   Joan McDowell

■ CONTENTS

INTRODUCTION

The history of the discovery of insulin in 1921 is one of trial and error, of personality clashes and of an Aberdonian receiving the Nobel prize. Without insulin the newly diagnosed diabetic child, teenager or young adult was faced with a slow, wasting disease which could only be treated by a starvation diet and led to an inevitable early death. The discovery of insulin offered a chance of life to those previously living without hope.

The first insulins produced were crude preparations of pancreatic extracts obtained from pigs and cattle. The insulin preparations were short-acting and while capable of keeping patients alive were unable to control their diabetes fully. This meant that patients had to suffer at least four painful injections each day. Subsequent research allowed the insulins to be prepared in different ways so that longer-acting preparations became available. Insulin however remained contaminated by other pancreatic peptide hormones and this could result in the development of insulin allergy. It was thought that if insulin could be 'cleaned up' and made more like human insulin then these problems could be overcome. In recent years, porcine and then beef insulins have been increasingly purified. More recently, synthetically produced insulins with the molecular structure identical to human insulin have become available.

About 20% of all patients with diabetes require insulin. Therefore for every 1000 patients on a general practice list, there will be 10–15 patients with diabetes of whom 3 or 4 will require insulin.

WHICH PATIENTS REQUIRE INSULIN?

Case Study 5.1

An 18-year-old male teenager presented to his GP with a 3-week history of thirst. He was drinking up to 2 litres of fizzy drinks per day. He had noticed that he was passing much more urine than normal and was having to get up through the night on at least three occasions to pass urine. During this period of time his weight had fallen by about 4 kg (half a stone). He had become increasingly tired and lethargic and had also noticed that his vision had become blurred. He also admitted to painful cracking of the foreskin and the presence of a white deposit on the penis. Glycosuria was confirmed as 2% and there was 3+++ of ketonuria using urine testing strips. The diagnosis was confirmed by measurement of plasma glucose of 23.0 mmol/l. The patient was referred immediately by telephone to the local consultant diabetologist, who arranged to see him the following day and insulin treatment was started.

The majority of patients with insulin-dependent diabetes mellitus (IDDM) will present as young adults under the age of 40 years. Patients presenting with IDDM typically give a short and dramatic history of polydipsia, polyuria and weight loss. The lack of insulin causes the blood glucose to rise, which acts as an osmotic diuretic causing polyuria and polydipsia. In an attempt to provide energy the body mobilises its glucose and fat reserves and in so doing, switches into ketone production (Ch. 1). This accounts for the massive weight loss, tiredness and lethargy. Left untreated, the patient would develop diabetic ketoacidosis and coma. Nowadays, this is less frequently seen due to heightened awareness of the early diabetic symptoms by health care workers.

The presence of glucose in the lens of the eye causes alteration in the shape of the lens and subsequent blurring of vision due to altered refraction. This corrects itself as blood glucose levels return to normal but may take up to 6 weeks before the blurring disappears. Newly diagnosed patients should be advised not to get their eyes tested for glasses for up to 3 months from diagnosis or until their diabetes is stable.

The presence of sugar in the urine can often cause penile thrush. Reducing glycosuria will discourage the growth of organisms. The patient however will also require appropriate antifungal treatment.

At the hospital clinic this man would be seen at his first visit by the consultant diabetologist, the dietitian and the diabetic nurse specialist (DNS). The consultant would perform a full physical examination and take blood samples for urea and electrolytes, liver function tests, full blood count and glycated haemoglobin. The dietitian would assess his current diet and initiate dietary changes in light of his history and estimated energy consumption. The DNS would start insulin therapy and home blood glucose monitoring (HBGM) and arrange to see him later in the day to continue his treatment. The young man would then enter a full education programme involving all the members of the health care team which may continue over several weeks or months (Ch. 10).

A further group of patients who require insulin therapy are those who have failed to respond to oral hypoglycaemic agents and diet. These will in general be older patients in whom drug therapy has failed to control the symptoms of hyperglycaemia.

There are also small numbers of patients who have diabetes secondary to diseases which damage the pancreas or diseases which result in increased resistance of the tissues to the actions of insulin (Ch. 1). These patients may also require insulin therapy.

WHAT ARE THE AIMS OF INSULIN THERAPY?

- first and foremost to preserve life
- to relieve the symptoms of hyperglycaemia—polydipsia, polyuria, lethargy and weight loss
- to restore 'normal metabolism'.

The first two aims are easily understood and apply to all patients regardless of age. The third aim is based on the belief that improved glycaemic control would protect patients from the long-term complications of diabetes. Several recent studies have clearly demonstrated that this is in fact the case (Hanssen et al 1992, The DCCT Research Group 1993).

It had been assumed that by replacing the insulin which is lacking, normal metabolism could be restored. It is now recognised that there are many subtle changes in the biochemistry of, for example, lipids, blood clotting and the connective tissues in patients with diabetes. Does insulin therapy correct these abnormalities? Should normal glycaemia be striven for or should the alleviation of symptoms suffice? Does good diabetic control really matter?

DOES GOOD DIABETIC CONTROL PREVENT DIABETIC COMPLICATIONS?

In order to attempt to answer the above question the Diabetes and Complications Trial was set up (The DCCT Research Group 1993). Nearly 1500 patients with insulin-dependent diabetes were recruited from 29 diabetic clinics across the USA. The patients were randomly allocated to receive up to 10 years' conventional or intensified treatment. Conventional therapy consisted of one or two daily injections of insulin and education about diet and exercise. Patients were reviewed every 3 months. The goals of conventional treatment included the absence of symptoms attributable to hyperglycaemia, absence of ketonuria, and maintenance of normal growth and ideal body weight. Intensified insulin treatment aimed for long-term near-normoglycaemia with at least four home blood glucose assessments a day, three insulin injections daily and monthly visits to a clinic with further advice freely available by telephone between clinics.

The trial was halted prematurely after patients had been followed up for periods ranging between 3 and 9 years. Patients in the intensively treated group maintained significantly better metabolic control throughout the study period. However, despite the intensive nature of their follow-up and treatment, only 5% of this group attained the goal of near-normoglycaemia throughout the study.

Nevertheless, the study dramatically demonstrated that tightening of diabetic control was associated with a significant reduction in the risks of developing diabetic complications or their progression. The 2% reduction in glycated haemoglobin of the intensively treated group of patients was associated with a 60% reduction in the risks of diabetic retinopathy, nephropathy and neuropathy. This improvement was apparent at all levels of metabolic control. In other words, a reduction in glycated haemoglobin from 16% to 14% was associated with the same improved outcome as a reduction from 10% to 8%. Patients with poorest control are clearly at the greatest risk of complications. Nevertheless, this study has implied that there is no threshold figure of glycated haemoglobin below which complications do not occur.

Other studies have however suggested that there may indeed be a 'safe' level for glycated haemoglobin and patients who maintain HbA$_1$ below such a threshold should be protected from microvascular complications (Krolewski et al 1995). Further work is required in order to clarify this important area.

The DCCT study has therefore confirmed the long-held belief of diabetic specialists, namely that the maintenance of tight metabolic control in patients is of long-term benefit. The study however has raised several questions regarding the intensity of treatment of patients. Financial and manpower restraints make it impossible to match the resources which were required in the DCCT to monitor patients and give continuing support and encouragement. Such intensive treatment and intrusive monitoring exert significant personal costs upon the patient with diabetes, who may find them intolerable. The patients may simply decide that it is not worth the trouble striving for good control.

Patients in the intensively treated group gained weight and experienced three times as many episodes of severe hypoglycaemia as the conventionally treated group. It should be remembered that the fear of severe hypoglycaemia concerns most young patients with IDDM more than the fear of complications in middle or late life.

A balance must be achieved between the objective of normoglycaemia on the one hand and the risk of hypoglycaemia and the inconvenience of intensive therapy on the other hand (Fig. 5.1). Most patients will be aiming for good diabetic control. However there are certain circumstances where this is more desirable than others.

Take for example the pregnant diabetic. Here the balance falls heavily in favour of tight glycaemic control preconceptually and during pregnancy (Fig. 5.1A), as this is a necessity for ensuring a successful outcome. Repeated hypoglycaemic episodes and the inconvenience of frequent blood glucose estimations and regular clinic visits are the price to be paid in order to tip the balance in the correct

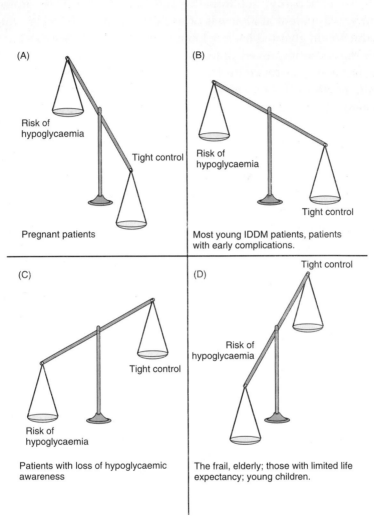

Fig. 5.1 IDDM: balance between the risk of hypoglycaemia and tight glycaemic control. (Based on Rizza R A, Greich J E, Haymond M W, Westland R E, Hall L D, Clemens A H, Service F S 1980 Control of blood sugar in insulin-dependent diabetes; comparison of an artificial endocrine pancreas, continuous subcutaneous insulin infusion, and intensified conventional insulin therapy. New England Journal of Medicine 303 (23):1313–1318, Table F1.

direction. On the other hand frail, elderly patients with limited life expectancy or those who are severely physically or mentally impaired cannot be expected to undergo the rigours required to achieve tight metabolic control (Fig. 5.1D).

However, for the vast majority of patients with IDDM the balance tilts to the side of maintaining tight diabetic control (Fig. 5.1B). The majority of these patients will have developed diabetes before the age of 40 years and would expect to live for many decades. Tight metabolic control offers these patients the best prospect of life which is not foreshortened and damaged by diabetic complications. These patients should follow an intensive diabetic regimen (Box 5.1) which requires the use of different insulin formulations and more than one injection of insulin per day. HBGM is essential to make appropriate alterations to insulin doses in response to these estimations. They should aim for a steady body weight at or near the desirable weight for their height. There should be absence of symptoms of diabetes with an incidence of mild hypoglycaemia which is acceptable to the patient. Pre-prandial blood glucose concentrations should be between 5 and 10 mmol/l and glycated haemoglobin levels close to normal.

Some discretion must be shown to young children (under the age of 10 years) in whom close diabetic control is difficult because of the variability of their eating habits and exercising patterns and their reluctance to cooperate with injections and HBGM. Intensive insulin therapy should be undertaken with extreme caution in children under the age of 7 years because hypoglycaemia may impair normal brain development, which is not complete until this age.

A similar relaxation of metabolic control may be required with patients who have lost the warning signs of impending hypoglycaemia (Fig. 5.1C). Over-zealous attempts to maintain close diabetic control

---

Box 5.1   Intensive diabetic regimen

- different formulations and/or multiple injections of insulin required
- insulin doses manipulated by patient according to results of HBGM
- steady body weight—at or near desirable weight (BMI <25)
- absence of diabetic symptoms with an incidence of hypoglycaemia acceptable to the patient
- blood glucose levels before meals between 5 and 10 mmol/l
- normal glycated haemoglobin levels

in these patients can result in an unacceptable incidence of severe hypoglycaemia.

INSULINS AVAILABLE FOR USE

Species

Bovine insulin differs from human insulin in three of its 51 amino acids, and is thus more likely to cause antibodies to be formed against it. Porcine insulin differs in only one amino acid residue (alanine in place of threonine). Insulins with a structure identical to human insulin are produced by two different methods.

Porcine insulin can be chemically altered by replacing the alanine amino acid with threonine (enzymically modified pro-insulin: emp insulin). Alternatively human insulin can be produced by introducing the gene for human insulin into bacteria or yeast (prb: proinsulin recombinant bacteria, or pyr: proinsulin recombinant yeast insulins, or ge: genetically engineered insulins). The organisms are cultured in huge vats and the insulin harvested and purified.

The early insulin preparations contained other pancreatic polypeptide hormones such as glucagon and also contained substantial amounts of the insulin precursor molecule, pro-insulin. In the 1970s highly purified porcine insulin was introduced and today the purity of all insulins is greatly improved.

Formulations

All commercial insulins are currently available in three broad types of formulation, classed according to their duration of action (Table 5.1).

First there is unmodified or soluble insulin which is short-acting and lasts for 5–8 hours when injected subcutaneously. The peak action of soluble insulin is 1–6 hours.

Then there are the intermediate-acting insulins (usually called isophane insulin in the UK or NPH insulin abroad). The action of this insulin is extended by complexing the insulin molecule with protamine (a large protein) and zinc. The mixture of neutral (or soluble) insulin with protamine and zinc was first invented by Hagedorn and the point where this complex is chemically formed is termed the 'isophane ratio'; hence the names, isophane or Neutral Protamine Hagedorn (NPH) insulin. The insulin-protamine-zinc complex is absorbed more slowly, extending its duration of action to between

Table 5.1 Insulin formulations and their duration of action. All insulins are human insulins, except for the Hypurin range, which is beef

Formulation	Examples	Total duration of action in hours		
		Onset	Duration	Peak
Soluble (neutral)	Actrapid	0.5	8	2.5–5
insulins	Velosulin	0.5	8	1–3
	Humulin S	0.5	5–7	1–3
	Hypurin Neutral	0.5–1	6–8	2–6
Isophane (NPH)	Insulatard	1.5	up to 24	4–12
insulins	Humulin I	1	18–20	2–8
	Hypurin isophane	within 2	18–24	6–12
Insulin Zinc	Monotard	2.5	2.5–22	7–15
suspensions	Humulin Lente	2.5	up to 24	4–16
	Hypurin Lente	2	up to 30	8–12
	Ultratard	4	4–28	8–24
	Humulin Zn	3	20–24	6–14

18 and 24 hours. The peak action of isophane insulins is usually 2–12 hours.

Finally there are the long-acting or lente insulins. If the insulin is mixed with zinc alone, it forms large insulin-zinc crystals which are slow to dissolve. Thus the action of crystalline zinc insulins can be extended beyond 24 hours and peak action does not begin for at least 4 hours.

Insulin regimens

Figure 5.2 shows the insulin concentrations in the blood of normal, nondiabetic subjects. It is evident that mealtimes are followed by immediate and sharp increases in insulin secretion as the pancreatic beta cells respond rapidly to rising blood levels of glucose. During the night and between meals there is a constant or basal secretion of insulin.

Conventional insulin therapy has attempted in several ways to simulate this physiological process. Figure 5.3 represents the once a day regimen which is perhaps only relevant for the frail, elderly diabetic. Although this regimen may be used infrequently in younger patients, those on once daily insulin injections will represent a significant proportion of the diabetic caseload of community nurses. It is obvious that this profile does not imitate normal physiology. It

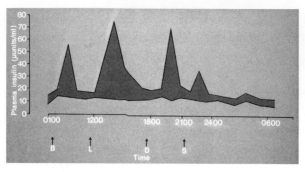

Fig. 5.2 Insulin concentrations in the blood of normal, nondiabetic subjects. Reprinted by permission of The New England Journal of Medicine, Copyright 1980, Massachusetts Medical Society, from Rizza R A et al, Control of blood sugar in insulin-dependent diabetes: comparison of an artificial endocrine pancreas, continuous subcutaneous insulin infusion, and intensified conventional insulin therapy. New England Journal of Medicine 303:1313–1318. Shaded areas represent one standard deviation above and below the mean for observations in six normal subjects. B denotes breakfast, L lunch, D dinner, S snack. Arrows indicate timing of insulin injections.

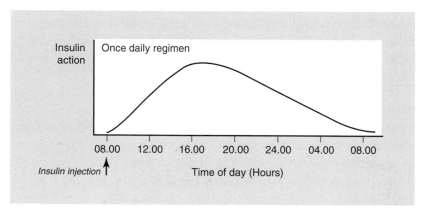

Fig. 5.3 Insulin therapy: once-daily regimen. Vertical arrow indicates insulin injection.

does however provide background insulin over 24 hours which is usually sufficient to prevent hyperglycaemia. Therefore for these patients breakfast can be taken prior to insulin injection. This has important implications for community nurses and the heavy case-load of weekend visiting.

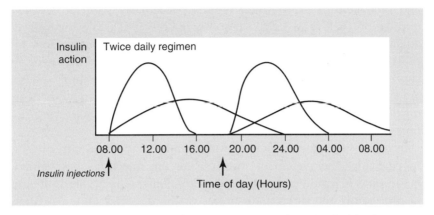

Fig. 5.4   Insulin therapy: twice-daily regimen. Arrows indicate insulin injections.

Figure 5.4 represents a conventional twice-daily regimen. The patient injects a mixture of short-acting and intermediate-acting insulins before breakfast and the evening meal. The profile of blood glucose levels produced by such a regimen differs significantly from physiological concentrations. Insulin is absorbed relatively slowly from the subcutaneous site and there are therefore no sharp, tall peaks of insulin secretion after meals. This inevitably means that patients become hyperglycaemic for an hour or so after eating. The profile between meals and during the night also does not simulate normal physiology. Insulin concentrations are higher than required during the evening but gradually fall throughout the night following the evening dose of insulin. This means that most patients on this regimen require an evening snack before retiring to bed, in order to prevent nocturnal hypoglycaemia.

Twice daily regimens for insulin administration have been the mainstay of treatment for patients with IDDM in this country for many years. Twice daily injections are convenient for most patients and fit well into the standard working day so that patients do not require to take their insulin with them to work. Some consultant diabetologists prefer to prescribe the soluble and intermediate insulins separately. This allows greater flexibility and allows fine adjustments to be made to the ratio of short- to longer-acting insulin.

It is well recognised that the accuracy of drawing up insulin is significantly reduced when patients are asked to draw up two insulins and mix them in the syringe. This is particularly so in an elderly population (Bell et al 1991, Kesson & Baillie 1981). The theoretical advantage of mixing individual insulins may therefore be lost in practice. For this reason other diabetologists prefer fixed mixtures of short- and intermediate-acting insulins (pre-mixed insulins). These are simpler to prescribe and use. Nowadays, the use of pen devices for the delivery of insulin is widespread and such devices use pre-mixed insulins.

In recent years, alternative insulin regimens have been introduced. In particular the system of multiple insulin injections has gained favour and is widely prescribed (Fig. 5.5). Patients inject short-acting insulin before the three main meals of the day and take a further injection of intermediate- or long-acting insulin usually before retiring to bed. The major advantage of this regimen is the flexibility which it provides. Mealtimes do not have to be adhered to rigidly. If a meal is delayed, the injection of soluble insulin can be withheld until half an hour before eating. Patients can anticipate altered activity (they may wish to take part in a sporting activity) or recognise that they will be eating more or less than usual. They can therefore make suitable adjustments to their insulin dosage. The use of insulin pen devices has allowed patients to carry their insulin with them in an acceptable form and to inject with relative convenience. Many people work complex shift systems and require the flexibility of a multiple injection regimen.

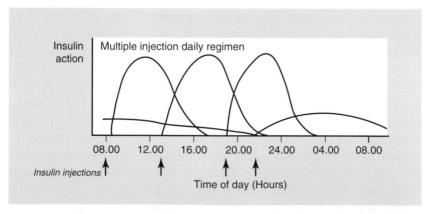

Fig. 5.5 Insulin therapy: multiple injection regimen. Arrows indicate insulin injections.

Continuous subcutaneous infusion of insulin (CSII)

A similar profile to Fig. 5.5 can be obtained using an insulin pump and continuous subcutaneous infusion of insulin. CSII, in theory, comes closest to mimicking the function of the pancreatic beta cell. A constant basal infusion of insulin is delivered by a pump device which is permanently connected to the skin with a 'butterfly' needle. The pump is capable of giving boluses of insulin prior to meals. However, the delivery of insulin to the subcutaneous site and not directly into the portal circulation means that the physiological peaks of insulin are not simulated. The system is not responsive to blood glucose concentrations and therefore cannot allow the fine adjustments in insulin delivery that can be made by the functioning beta cell.

CSII is rarely used except in some diabetic centres where there is particular expertise. Pumps are expensive and require careful supervision by the diabetic consultant. Ketoacidosis can develop rapidly in patients on CSII if they become ill or if the pump fails. This is because there is no subcutaneous depot of insulin to act as a reserve. 24-hour access to clinic personnel is therefore essential. There is also a large psychological component in wearing a pump 24 hours a day and many patients find this unacceptable. Pump therapy has therefore not proved popular in this country and few general practices will have experience of patients on pumps.

Which insulin to use?

The choice of insulin will clearly depend upon the type of regimen which has been determined in consultation with the patient. The actual source of insulin is arbitrary, although patients who are forbidden by their religion or creed to consume animal products may often use biosynthetic insulin only. Most religions however will accept animal insulins in the absence of any suitable alternative.

It should be remembered that there is great variability in the absorption of insulin from the subcutaneous site. Insulin is absorbed most rapidly from the abdominal wall, then from the arms and most slowly from thighs and buttocks (Galloway et al 1981). Alterations in skin blood flow will also affect the rate of insulin absorption. Increased blood flow due to exercise or raised skin temperature will result in more rapid insulin absorption. Other variables such as subcutaneous fat thickness and insulin dose also influence insulin pharmacokinetics, not to mention poor injection techniques (Sindelka et al 1994). It should therefore not come as a surprise to find that the same dose of insulin will have differing effects on the same patient from day to day. It is tempting to make subtle alterations in insulin doses and ratios of soluble to isophane insulin in an attempt to improve diabetic control. Normal day-to-day fluctuations in the response to insulin should however be considered and daily dose alterations are not encouraged. The routine adjustment of insulin dose is discussed later in the chapter.

Human insulin and loss of hyoglycaemic awareness

At an inquest in England in 1989 into the sudden death of a young diabetic patient, a forensic chemist provided information which implicated human insulin in the death, which may have been due to severe hypoglycaemia. Much has subsequently been written in the popular press and presented on our television screens regarding the reputed dangers of human insulin products.

Many patients have reported alteration or loss of hypoglycaemic awareness after changing to human insulin and a group of physicians in Switzerland reported that the symptoms of hypoglycaemia in their patients on human insulin were reduced and the incidence of severe hypoglycaemic attacks was subsequently increased (Teuscher & Berger 1987). These findings have not been confirmed in most other countries and at present there is no consensus reached regarding the effects of human insulin on hypoglycaemia.

There are two main reasons why patients may experience loss of hypoglycaemic awareness: these are tight metabolic control and autonomic neuropathy.

Strict control of diabetes is recognised to impair perception of the onset of hypoglycaemia. In the well-controlled patient, as the body becomes accustomed to normal blood glucose levels, the threshold for the release of the counter-regulatory hormones becomes lower and patients do not experience the symptoms of hypoglycaemia until the blood glucose concentrations are well within the hypoglycaemic range. Indeed the patients may not recognise hypoglycaemia until it is too late and cognition is already impaired by severe hypoglycaemia.

There is also evidence that a recent hypoglycaemic event results in impaired perception of subsequent hypoglycaemia; hypoglycaemia begets hypoglycaemia (Heller & Cryer 1991).

Some patients will lose the warning symptoms of hypoglycaemia if they develop autonomic neuropathy. Hypoglycaemia in these patients fails to result in stimulation of the sympathetic nervous system and there is no release of adrenalin in response to low glucose levels. Thus patients with autonomic neuropathy will lack most of the early warning signs of hypoglycaemia. This form of hypoglycaemic unawareness tends to develop slowly and is not usually evident until the patient has been diabetic for at least 15 years (Frier 1993).

At present there is insufficient evidence to support the suggestion that the awareness of hypoglycaemia is reduced by human insulin, nor that there is a greater incidence of either severe or fatal hypoglycaemia with human insulin. The major causes of reduced hypoglycaemic awareness are duration of the diabetes and recent strict glycaemic control. If a patient reports altered or reduced awareness of hypoglycaemia following the introduction of human insulin it is important in the first instance to make sure that the metabolic control is not too strict. Doctors and community nurses should however remain receptive to their patients' views and any patient who feels unhappy with human insulin or who experiences hypoglycaemic-related problems should be permitted to revert to animal insulin preparations.

Insulin treatment in the elderly

The use of insulin in NIDDM is more fully discussed in Chapter 4. The world's elderly population, aged 65 years and older, is currently growing at a rate of 2.5%/year, considerably faster than the overall population. The fastest growing age segment of all is the very elderly, defined as those over 80 years. Eight developed countries now have very elderly populations numbering greater than 1 million and six more nations will share this statistic by the year 2020 (Torrey et al, US Bureau of the Census 1987). The number of very elderly people with diabetes will correspondingly increase and impose a considerable burden upon the resources of the community health care team. Insulin therapy in the elderly should not be embarked upon lightly and several factors should be taken into consideration before instigating such treatment.

There is little value in attempting to achieve tight metabolic control in a patient who has limited life expectancy. The complications of diabetes take many years to develop and therefore may not contribute significantly to that patient's morbidity or mortality. Life expectancy for patients of varying ages is shown in Table 5.2. When judging the potential value of insulin therapy in the elderly it is important to treat all patients as individuals. An assessment of the 'biological age' of a patient is often made. Thus an active, alert and physically fit 75-year-old may cope with and gain greater benefit from insulin therapy than a frail, forgetful 65-year-old patient who has had a cerebrovascular accident.

The elderly with diabetes may have several physical problems which directly affect their ability to inject insulin and monitor control. Poor eyesight due to cataract formation or senile macular degeneration is common in this age group and will clearly impair the diabetic patient's ability to administer and monitor insulin treatment accurately. One survey of insulin-treated elderly patients with diabetes attending a UK hospital clinic found that 51% had visual acuities of 6/18 or worse in one or both eyes (Pegg et al 1991). Tremor and poor muscular coordination also afflict this age group and there is some evidence that these muscular problems are more common in an ageing diabetic population if compared to non-diabetics (Lord et al 1993). Other problems, including strokes, rheumatism, memory loss or Parkinson's disease, may further impair function in the elderly.

The ability to alter lifestyle and accept change can be compromised in this age group. Similarly, their ability to acquire new knowledge may be defective and many elderly patients are unable to make the

Table 5.2 Expectation of life for the general population of the UK (1991–1993)

Age (years)	Scotland[†]		England and Wales[*]	
	Males	Females	Males	Females
65	13.3	16.8	14.3	18.1
70	10.4	13.4	11.2	14.5
75	8.0	10.4	8.6	11.2
80	6.1	7.8	6.5	8.4
85	4.6	5.7	4.8	6.1

[†]Figures for Scotland from the Registrar General for Scotland.
[*]Figures for England and Wales from the Government Actuary's Dept.

changes necessary to allow themselves to look after their insulin treatment. Patients therefore become dependent upon relatives or community staff with a resulting deterioration in their independence and self-esteem. In one survey of elderly patients' status 2 years after starting insulin treatment it was found that insulin was regularly administered by a third party in more than 60% of patients. Of those who were self-injecting, almost one third were doing so incorrectly and a large minority were also monitoring urine or blood inaccurately (Elgrably et al 1991). This study also found that almost 40% of elderly patients gained little or no benefit from any of the educational methods used. It is therefore not surprising that another survey of patients attending a London teaching hospital found serious deficiencies in the knowledge and management skills of the elderly patient on insulin. Almost half of the elderly patients were unaware of any symptoms of hyperglycaemia and a similar proportion would take potentially dangerous action in the event of a foot injury. 25% of this population had required hospital attendance for the treatment of hypoglycaemia in the previous year (Pegg et al 1991).

Hypoglycaemia is common in the elderly patient treated with insulin (Elgrably et al 1991, Rump et al 1987). This may partly be due to poor understanding by the patient, and in particular a lack of knowledge or awareness of the symptoms of hypoglycaemia. In addition, the elderly patient may be more susceptible to alterations in cognitive function in response to reductions in blood glucose (Meneilly et al 1994). Other physiological factors are also of prime importance. Hypoglycaemia results from the presence of excess insulin in the circulation and recovery from hypoglycaemia will occur as the insulin levels fall. The body is able to respond to hypoglycaemia by stimulating the secretion of other hormones which can counteract the actions of insulin. These hormones, glucagon, adrenalin, and to a lesser extent growth hormone and cortisol, are termed the counter-regulatory hormones. Any impairment of the body's ability to metabolise insulin or impairment of the counter-regulatory responses will increase the risks of severe or fatal hypoglycaemia. There is good evidence that the elderly have both impairment of insulin clearance and faulty counter-regulatory responses to hypoglycaemia (Marker et al 1992, Meneilly et al 1994). The elderly are more likely to live alone and their isolation may delay receiving assistance to treat hypoglycaemia. Hence hypoglycaemia ought to be avoided.

Case Study 5.2

A 75-year-old woman has had diabetes for 20 years. Initially she was treated by diet alone. After 5 years she was started on the oral hypoglycaemic, gliclazide. She responded well to this treatment. However over the last 3 years her diabetic control has been poorer and the dose of gliclazide has gradually been increased to maximum. The dietitian confirms that she is complying with a diabetic diet. Never significantly overweight, her weight has been gradually falling during the past 2–3 years. She has significant symptoms of polydipsia and polyuria and rises through the night on three or four occasions to pass urine. She suffers from angina and has required treatment for high blood pressure for many years. She complains of cramps in her legs at night and her feet are always cold. She has bilateral cataracts and her vision is poor; she is unable to read and finds watching television difficult. She lives by herself and although she appears to cope well at home, she does admit that she is more forgetful nowadays.

This patient now requires insulin therapy. She has symptoms of hyperglycaemia and is losing weight. Although she does not admit it, she is probably more tired and lethargic than normal. She however attributes these symptoms to old age. She has ischaemic heart disease, peripheral vascular disease and hypertension. Her cognitive function is impaired and she is unable to benefit from written information sheets. She may well be unable to learn the new skills required of the insulin-taking diabetic and her poor vision may also prevent her from self-monitoring or injecting. Hypoglycaemia should also be avoided in patients with ischaemic heart disease, when arrhythmias can occur.

The aim of treatment in such a patient should be to relieve the symptoms of hyperglycaemia without striving for tight metabolic control. A steady body weight should be aimed for even if this weight is not ideal. There should be a minimum of HBGMs since the blood glucose level is relatively unimportant. The simplest possible insulin regimen should be adopted and this will usually involve a single daily injection of an isophane insulin prior to breakfast. In this particular patient's case the insulin might be administered by a community nurse who can measure the blood glucose weekly. This less intensive regimen is shown in Box 5.2.

Box 5.2   Less intensive diabetic regimen

- simplest possible insulin regimen (usually 1 injection per day)
- the minimum of HBGM
- a steady body weight even if BMI >25
- freedom of symptoms of hyperglycaemia
- glycosuria of 0.5% or less
- blood glucose levels below 20 mmol/l acceptable

PANCREATIC AND ISLET CELL
TRANSPLANTATION FOR IDDM

From time to time health care professionals may be asked by their patients with IDDM whether they can be cured by pancreatic or islet cell transplantation. It is important therefore that some background information is available to the primary health care team on this subject.

The primary restriction to pancreatic transplantation is the requirement to treat patients with immunosuppressive therapy following such a procedure. Immunosuppression is not without risk since it reduces the patient's defence against infection and the development of malignancy. Most clinicians would judge that the risk of immunosuppression for pancreatic transplantation alone is not justified. Pancreatic transplantation in the UK is therefore restricted to those patients with diabetes who are in need of renal transplants and would be receiving immunosuppressive drugs as a matter of course.

The outcome of pancreatic surgery is often disappointing. Despite 15–20 years' experience in some centres, 30–35% of transplanted glands fail during the first year and more than half will have failed by 5 years (Abecassis & Corry 1993, Sutherland 1992).

Since pancreatic transplantation is confined in this country to patients receiving renal transplants, it means that patients who undergo such surgery are also the patients who have well-established diabetic complications. Pancreatic transplantation can only be expected to halt the progression of these complications rather than cure them. Unfortunately there is little evidence that such surgery does arrest or delay the complications of diabetes (Robertson 1992).

The results for islet cell transplantation are even less encouraging.

Despite many years of research and many attempts to transplant islet cells, relief of dependence on insulin has hardly ever been achieved. It has proved difficult to obtain sufficient numbers of cells for transplantation and to protect them from subsequent rejection. New methods of harvesting the cells and of protection against the immune system are required before this procedure can become a clinical reality.

NURSE PRESCRIBING

Nurses have always been nervous about insulin dose adjustment from both a professional and legal aspect. Nurse prescribing, although first proposed in 1986, was not given royal assent until 1992 (Cumberlege 1986). An advisory group reported that there were three areas in which nurses could prescribe after completing further education in the subject (Crown 1989).

The first area is where community nurses would sign their own prescriptions for products listed on the Nurses' Formulary. In addition to this many nurses, e.g. continence advisers, practice nurses and school nurses, supply products within a group protocol. Lastly there are those nurses who 'adjust timing and dosages of medicines'. In community care this would include palliative care nurses and community psychiatric nurses.

From this it would appear that DNSs, after suitable education, will in future be professionally covered for those aspects of their role which they currently undertake. This usually includes the initiation and alteration of insulin therapy and adjustment of insulin doses. While currently DNSs do not appear to have prescribing rights under law, it is common custom and practice. So saying, they do not assume this role until after appropriate education and training by the hospital consultant.

It is therefore essential that those undertaking insulin dose adjustment as part of the extended role of the nurse acquire the necessary knowledge and supervised training (Cradock 1993). Hence it is not normally considered within the remit of the community nurse who may only attend one or two patients on insulin on an irregular basis.

Insulin dose adjustment

The patient with diabetes who has been instructed on insulin dose adjustment by the DNS may find it difficult to obtain further advice from other health care professionals. This may be because the health care professionals may not have sufficient experience. Knowledge, competence and confidence are essential for undertaking insulin dose adjustment.

Insulin doses vary according to type of insulin, frequency of injections, proposed exercise, planned diet and any other underlying illness or stress. While the GP prescribes the bottle of insulin, the dose to be administered is variable. However, patients seldom self-adjust safely and appropriately. It is therefore advocated that patients should be specifically taught and audited on their response to self-adjustment of insulin. Unless this is done, self-adjustment should not be encouraged (Gill & Redmond 1991).

So saying, the principle of insulin dose adjustment is fairly easy to explain. Included here are some general guidelines which should allow the PHCT to give simple advice and reassurance to the patients. This will not make the PHCT competent at insulin dose adjustment. The following are therefore principles for ROUTINE insulin dose adjustment—that is adjustments for the well patient and not for the ill patient with diabetes who is needing frequent, large increases of insulin. These latter patients should be referred immediately to the DNS or Hospital Clinic.

A prerequisite for insulin dose adjustment is HBGM (Ch. 7). The blood glucose test should be performed prior to food and insulin. Blood glucose levels are affected by many things (Box 5.3).

If a patient's blood glucose levels are high then try to find a cause for this before considering insulin dose increases. Some suitable questions to ask are:

- Has the patient some other illness, e.g. a chest infection?
- Is there some underlying stress factor which is raising the blood glucose profile?
- How much exercise does the patient usually take and has this altered recently?
- Has the patient been indulging in too many dietary indiscretions?
- Are other medical treatments, e.g. steroid therapy, interfering with diabetic control?

Only if there is no other explanation should routine insulin dose adjustment be considered.

Box 5.3   Cause of high and low blood glucose levels

Cause of high blood glucose levels

- not enough insulin
- not enough exercise
- too much food
- stress
- any other illness
- erratic absorption of insulin
- other medication

Cause of low blood glucose levels

- too much insulin
- too much/unexpected exercise not accommodated for
- not enough food including delaying or missing a meal
- alcohol
- recovering from an illness
- erratic absorption of insulin

Erratic blood glucose profiles should not be treated. A profile which swings between high and low results is best left alone. Questions may be asked regarding injection sites, timing of injections, doses being injected, experiences of hypoglycaemia, etc. Injection sites should be inspected for any lipohypertrophy and if any is present then those areas should be avoided until the lipohypertrophy recedes. Erratic profiles which cause concern should be referred to the DNS or hospital clinic for more in-depth assessment and necessary changes.

Routine insulin dose adjustment is usually considered when there are three sets of results to evaluate. As patients with diabetes may monitor only twice a week then this would mean that routine adjustment may only be considered every 10 days.

In setting goals for patients it is important that these are realistic, short-term and achievable. Hence if a patient has blood glucose levels constantly around 13–15 mmol/l it is more realistic to set the goal initially as 10–13 mmol/l. Once the blood glucose profile is between 10 and 13 mmol/l then the next goal could be set as 8–10 mmol/l and so on.

Working on three sets of results, the patient is taught to increase the relevant insulin by 2 units only. The RELEVANT insulin is that insulin which has been acting to give the high blood glucose result. In other words, a blood glucose REFLECTS the previous insulin dose.

Case Study 5.3

A patient is taking 16 units of insulin before breakfast and 14 units before evening meal. The patient is aiming for blood glucose levels of 8–10 mmol/l. The patient is keeping to his diet, is taking no other medication, has not altered his exercise nor is he experiencing any undue stress. His blood glucose results on three occasions are:

Before breakfast (mmol/l)	Before evening meal (mmol/l)
9	13
8.4	12
9.6	13.5

This patient has three sets of results above 10 mmol/l before his evening meal, which reflects the breakfast dose of insulin. The breakfast insulin dose should therefore be increased the following day by two units to 18 units.

Once it is increased, the patient would be advised to continue monitoring and wait until he had acquired a further three sets of results before continuing to increase his insulin dose. Only one insulin dose should be adjusted at any one time. In this way, a high blood glucose is 'tickled' down and is not decreased rapidly.

Patients who have consistently low blood glucose results can also decrease the relevant insulin using the same principle.

This protocol for insulin dose adjustment is not relevant for those patients on a once-daily injection of a long-acting insulin. Such insulins have long half-lives which means that insulin can accumulate in the circulation and cause prolonged hypoglycaemia. Any erratic control with these patients should be referred to the DNS or hospital clinic. Often these patients are elderly and supervised by the community nurse and the risks of hypoglycaemia far outweigh any immediate benefit of reducing a blood glucose level.

Those patients who practise self-adjustment should be encouraged to use the knowledge that they have gained. Health care professionals who know the underlying principles of routine insulin dose adjustment can support their patients.

INJECTION TECHNIQUES AND EQUIPMENT

It is now recognised that surgical spirit is unnecessary to clean the skin prior to injecting insulin. The absence of surgical spirit not only removes the 'sting' from the injection but also reduces the chances of the patient acquiring leather-like skin in later years! It is still important however that hands and skin are clean to the naked eye prior to the injection.

A survey into whether it is necessary to inject air into the insulin bottle prior to drawing up the injection was inconclusive in its results (Richmond 1991). It was noted that although most professionals and patients are taught to inject air into the insulin bottle prior to drawing up the injection, they did not all practise this. While some people experience no problems others have found that the creation of a vacuum within the bottle causes air bubbles to be drawn into the syringe. Therefore until this is further researched it would seem reasonable to continue with the practice of injecting air into the bottle prior to drawing up insulin.

The recommended angle for injecting insulin has altered over recent years. The objective is for insulin to be injected into subcutaneous tissue and not into the deeper muscle layer. With the introduction of shorter length needles a perpendicular approach is now favoured for injecting. However in thin patients, insulin may still be injected into the underlying muscle using this technique. For this reason it has been suggested that thin patients should grasp a skinfold, insert the needle at a 45 degree angle then release the skinfold before injecting the insulin (Engstrom 1994). Assessing the patient's skinfolds will determine whether a perpendicular approach or one at 45 degrees will reach subcutaneous tissue.

It remains important to rotate the injection sites to prevent lipohypertrophy occurring. Lipohypertrophy can cause erratic absorption of insulin. Different sites have different absorption rates. Community nurses will be familiar with the patient who has their left arm exposed for their insulin injection every morning! While rotating sites is important, in this instance it would probably be wise to move to the right arm for a short while before attempting to introduce the other areas.

Often community nurses are asked to assume responsibility for insulin injections for elderly patients who are losing their eyesight. The patients themselves may wish to remain as independent as possible. In this instance it is worth investigating the various pen devices to see if any are suitable for the patient to use. Alternatively, if the patient remains competent in the injection technique, there is no reason why he/she could not be left with a preloaded syringe for injection later. This would afford the patient some degree of independence from community nursing services (Royal College of Nursing 1991).

After injecting, the needle can be safely removed using the BD safeclip device which is available on prescription. The syringe can be disposed of, either in a sharps box or else in an opaque hard plastic container with the lid screwed on and securely taped, before placing in a disposal bin.

Although insulin syringes are now available on prescription, the needles required for the pen devices are not. It is considered quite safe for disposable syringes to be re-used for a period of 7 days and any needle need only be changed when it becomes blunt (Pickup & Williams 1991).

CONCLUSION

There are various insulin types available on the market. There is no insulin which is more suitable than others for patients. Recent publicity around the reported loss of hypoglycaemic warning signs associated with human insulin has not been supported by research. However, where a patient complains of a loss of warning signs and believes this is due to human insulin then he/she should be changed back to their previous animal insulin.

General Practitioners prescribe an insulin bottle but the dose is very variable. To achieve maximum diabetic control, patients are taught how to adjust their own insulin doses. However it is important that those patients doing so are audited and supported in this. Nurse prescribing is becoming a reality but for the majority of community nurses, insulin dose adjustment will not become part of their role.

Insulin injections should be delivered to the subcutaneous tissues. Syringes and needles should be disposed of safely.

REFERENCES

Abecassis M, Corry R J 1993 An update on pancreas transplantation. Advances in Surgery:163–188

Bell D S, Clements R S Jr, Perentesis G, Roddam R, Wagenknecht L 1991 Dosage accuracy of self-mixed vs premixed insulin. Archives of Internal Medicine 151:2265–2269

Cumberlege J 1986 Neighbourhood nursing: a focus for care. DHSS, London

Cradock S 1993 Adjusting insulin dose. Community Outlook 3:7:18–20

Crown J 1989 Report of the advisory group on nurse prescribing. Department of Health, London

The DCCT Research Group 1993 The effect of intensive treatment of diabetes on the development and progression of long-term complications in insulin-dependent diabetes mellitus. New England Journal of Medicine 329:977–986

Elgrably F, Costagliola D, Chwalow A J, Varenne P, Slama G, Tchobroutsky G 1991 Initiation of insulin treatment after 70 years of age: patient status 2 years later. Diabetic Medicine 8:773–777

Engstrom L 1994 Technique of insulin injection: is it important? Practical Diabetes 11: 1:39

Frier B M 1993 Hypoglycaemia unawareness. In: Frier B M, Fisher B M Hypoglycaemia and diabetes. Hodder & Stoughton, London

Galloway J A, Spradlin C T, Nelson R L, Wentworth S M, Davidson J A, Swarner J L 1981 Factors influencing the absorption, serum insulin concentration, and blood glucose responses after injections of regular insulin and various insulin mixtures. Diabetes Care 4:366–376

Gill G V, Redmond S 1991 Self-adjustment of insulin: an educational failure? Practical Diabetes 8:4:142–143

Hanssen K F, Bangtad H-J, Brinchmann-Hansen O, Dahl-Jorgensen K 1992 Blood glucose control and diabetic microvascular complications: long-term effects of near-normoglycaemia. Diabetic Medicine 9:697–705

Heller S R, Cryer P E 1991 Reduced neuroendocrine and symptomatic responses to subsequent hypoglycaemia after one episode of hypoglycaemia in nondiabetic humans. Diabetes 40:223–226

Kesson C M, Baillie G R 1981 Do diabetic patients inject accurate doses of insulin? (letter) Diabetes Care 4:333

Krolewski A S, Laffel L M B, Krolewski M, Quinn M, Warram J H 1995 Glycosylated hemoglobin and the risk of microalbuminuria in patients with insulin-dependent diabetes mellitus. New England Journal of Medicine 332:1251–1255

Lord S R, Caplan G A, Colagiuri R, Colagiuri S, Ward J A 1993 Sensori-motor function in older persons with diabetes. Diabetic Medicine 10:614–618

Marker J C, Cryer P E, Clutter W E 1992 Attenuated glucose recovery from hypoglycaemia in the elderly. Diabetes 41:671–678

Meneilly G S, Cheung E, Tuokko H 1994 Altered responses to hypoglycaemia of healthy elderly people. Journal of Clinical Endocrinology and Metabolism 78:1341–1348

Pegg A, Fitzgerald F, Wise D, Singh B M, Wise P H 1991 A community-based study of diabetes-related skills and knowledge in elderly patients with insulin-requiring diabetes. Diabetic Medicine 8:778–781

Pickup J C, Williams G 1991 Insulin injection treatment for insulin-dependent diabetic patients. In: Pickup J C, Williams G (eds) Textbook of diabetes. Blackwell Scientific, Oxford

Richmond J 1991 Injecting air into insulin bottles—necessary or not? Diabetic Nursing 2:2:6–7

Rizza R A, Greich J E, Haymond M W, Westland R E, Hall L D, Clemens A H, Service F S 1980 Control of blood sugar in insulin dependent diabetes; comparison of an artificial endocrine pancreas, continuous subcutaneous insulin infusion, and intensified conventional insulin therapy. New England Journal of Medicine 303 (23):1313–1318

Robertson R P 1992 Pancreatic and islet transplantation for diabetes—cures or curiosities? New England Journal of Medicine 327:1861–1866

Royal College of Nursing of the United Kingdom Diabetes Nursing Forum 1991 Guidelines on pre-mixing/pre-loading of insulin by community nurses for patients to give at a later time. RCN Diabetes Nursing Forum, London

Rump A, Stahl M, Caduff F, Berger W 1987 173 cases of insulin-induced hypoglycaemia admitted to hospital. Deutsche Medizinische Wochenschrift 112:1110–1116

Sindelka G, Heinemann L, Berger M, Frenck W, Chantelau E 1994 Effect of insulin concentration, subcutaneous fat thickness and skin temperature on subcutaneous insulin absorption in healthy subjects. Diabetologia 37:377–380

Sutherland D E R 1992 Pancreatic transplantation: state of the art. Transplantation Proceedings 24:762–766

Teuscher A and Berger W G 1987 Hypoglycaemia unawareness in diabetics transferred from beef/porcine insulin to human insulin. Lancet II:382–385

Torrey B B, Kinsella K, Taeuber C M (eds) 1987 An aging world. US Bureau of the Census International Population Reports Series P-95 No. 78. U.S. Government Printing Service, Washington DC

Dietary advice

June Gordon

DIET AND DIABETES—FROM PAST TO PRESENT

Diabetes is one of the oldest diseases known to man, and historically diet has been linked with both its cause and cure. For centuries little was known about the disease and the search for a dietary cure relied on trial and error. When it was discovered that the urine of diabetic patients was sweet, it was thought that the diet should be rich in carbohydrate to make up for these urinary losses. An alternative view was that the body could not cope with carbohydrate foods and that they should therefore be avoided.

Dietary advice fluctuated between the two extremes of high carbohydrate 'cures' (based on skimmed milk and oatmeal) to low carbohydrate diets of meat and boiled vegetables. Even after the discovery of insulin in 1921, carbohydrate restriction was advocated.

Today diet still plays a central role in the treatment of diabetes, but the composition has changed considerably and recommendations are now in line with those for a healthy diet for the general population.

THE IMPORTANCE OF DIET

Diet is the cornerstone of treatment and for many it is the only form of treatment required. Approximately 80% of patients are non-insulin-dependent and controlled on either diet alone or diet and oral hypo-glycaemic agents. The remaining 20% are insulin-dependent and controlled on diet and insulin injections.

The role of the nurse in providing dietary advice

Because of the central role of diet in management, the British Diabetic Association advises that all newly diagnosed patients receive indi-vidualised dietary advice and regular updates from a State Registered Dietitian. There may be a delay before the patient has access to a dietitian and the nurse may be required to give first-line advice. Suit-able advice to give to a newly diagnosed patient is given in Box 6.1.

The frequency of visits to a dietitian will depend on available resources. Some hospital and community dietetic departments produce GP packs which help nurses give out appropriate information to patients, and some run training courses for local primary health care staff. Whatever the situation it is worth making contact with the local nutrition and dietetic department as good communication can only benefit the patient as well as ensure consistency of advice. Nurses can play a vital role in providing general dietary guidance as backup to the more specific advice given by the dietitian, as well as reinforcing this advice and identifying specific situations where more detailed information is required.

Box 6.1   Initial dietary advice suitable to give to a patient prior to their appointment with a dietitian

1. Quench thirst with water or sugar-free drinks, e.g. diet lemonades and diet cola drinks.
2. Have regular meals, avoiding fried or very sugary foods.
3. Eat plenty of vegetables with cereal, bread, pasta, potato, rice or chapati as the main part of the meal.
4. Have meat, cheese, eggs as a small part of the meal. Try fish, chicken and pulses as alternatives.

The BDA produce a leaflet, 'Food and diabetes—just a beginning', which may be useful as preliminary advice.

THE AIMS OF DIETARY TREATMENT

The immediate treatment aim for diabetes is to control hyperglycaemia, but the ultimate aim is to allow the person to lead as normal a life as possible, in good health, and for most patients to achieve a weight as close as possible to the 'ideal'. Controlling total energy intake and encouraging physical activity are essential parts of the treatment.

The overall aims of dietary treatment are summarised in Box 6.2.

BACKGROUND TO THE CURRENT DIETARY RECOMMENDATIONS

Dietary advice prior to the 1980s centred on carbohydrate restriction as the only means of controlling blood glucose levels. People were advised to limit their intake of carbohydrate foods such as bread, potatoes, rice, pasta and cereals and to fill up on foods such as meat, cheese, eggs, cream and butter. This resulted in a diet low in carbohydrate, but high in fat. Research in the 1970s (Brunzell et al 1974, Simpson et al 1979) showed that high carbohydrate diets could actually improve diabetic control, providing the carbohydrate was in a complex, high-fibre form. Studies were also beginning to show that reducing fat intake in nondiabetic patients resulted in reduced morbidity from cardiovascular disease (Miettinen et al 1977). This led researchers to ask whether the high fat diet could be contributing to the increased risk of heart disease in patients with diabetes.

As a result of this research the British Diabetic Association (BDA) published dietary recommendations for diabetes in 1982 (British

---

Box 6.2   The aims of dietary treatment

1. Abolish the primary symptoms of diabetes.
2. Achieve and maintain an agreed target body weight.
3. Maintain blood glucose and lipids at as near normal levels as possible.
4. Minimise the risk of hypoglycaemia in those treated with oral hypoglycaemic agents or with insulin.
5. Minimise the long-term macrovascular and microvascular complications of diabetes.

Diabetic Association Nutrition Subcommittee 1982) which marked the abandoning of the traditional low carbohydrate 'diabetic diet'. This policy statement was considered to be a radical document, but it was followed by the introduction of almost identical policies by Diabetes Associations in many other countries. It was also very similar to nutritional guidelines published for the general United Kingdom population (Department of Health and Social Security COMA report 1984) and of the World Health Organization (James et al, WHO 1988) for Europe. This had positive implications in that people with diabetes were no longer being advised to follow a 'special diabetic diet', but instead to follow healthy eating guidelines recommended for the general population.

In 1992, the BDA updated their recommendations (British Diabetic Association Nutrition Subcommittee 1992a). These reinforce the general principles of the 1982 recommendations, but include some changes in emphasis as a result of new scientific evidence available. Total energy, carbohydrate, fat and protein intakes and meal patterns are all now considered in relation to diabetic control (Box 6.3).

TRANSLATING RECOMMENDATIONS INTO PRACTICAL ADVICE

The scientific evidence for the effect of diet on diabetes needs to be translated into practical guidance which can be used directly with the patient. A simple, flexible approach is required and counselling skills should be used to motivate the individual to make positive and achievable dietary changes. Not all patients will be able (or willing) to achieve all dietary goals and a balance should be found between what is acceptable, achievable and beneficial to that patient.

It is worth noting that the majority of patients are non-insulin-dependent and present over the age of 40 years. This means that their eating habits are already well established and change may be difficult. Some may have been diabetic for more than 20 years and may remember the initial dietary advice given to them at diagnosis. This change from a low to a high carbohydrate diet may be difficult to accept, especially if the patient is in the habit of weighing foods (which a minority of patients do still practise). Many patients with diabetes consider diet to be the most difficult and traumatic part of treatment and this is a point worth remembering when giving dietary advice.

Box 6.3   Summary of nutritional recommendations for diabetes (BDA 1992a)

1. Reducing energy intake remains the most important aim for those who are overweight.
2. Carbohydrate should make up 50–55% of daily energy intake. Most of this should be in the form of complex carbohydrate foods naturally high in dietary fibre.
3. Regular meals are important. All meals and snacks should contain carbohydrate.
4. A target of 30 g of fibre (or 18–20 g of non-starch polysaccharides) is advised, with emphasis on soluble fibre.
5. Up to 25 g (1 oz) added sucrose may be included, providing it is part of a high fibre, low fat diet.
6. Reducing fat intake to 30–35% of daily energy intake is important in aiming to reduce the incidence of coronary heart disease. Saturated fats should contribute no more than 10% of energy, and 10% should be polyunsaturated and 10–15% monounsaturated.
7. Cholesterol intake should not be greater than 300 mg per day. This should be achieved automatically by reducing saturated fat to 10% of energy.
8. Protein should make up 10–15% of energy. Reducing protein intake may help to slow down the progression of nephropathy.
9. Salt intake should not be greater than 6 g per day.
10. Special diabetic products should not be recommended.

Although the principles of the diet for diabetes are similar to those for a healthy diet for the rest of the population, it still represents a significant deviation from the typical UK diet. If the whole family are supportive and are prepared to make changes towards better eating habits, it can help the patient to follow the appropriate dietary advice. Diabetes should be seen as the catalyst for change which can ultimately improve the future health of the family.

PUTTING THE RECOMMENDATIONS INTO PRACTICE

Energy

In dietary terms, the energy content of the diet in relation to the energy requirement probably has the greatest influence on long-term diabetes control. If the amount of energy from food is greater than the amount the body requires, the excess will be stored as fat and obesity can result. This can make diabetes difficult to control because the body tissues become more resistant to the action of insulin. Weight reduction will improve diabetic control because as adipose tissue is lost, the insulin that is being produced will be able to work more effectively. The aim is that most patients with diabetes should consume the appropriate amount of energy to keep their weight within the ideal range.

Carbohydrate

The recommendation is that at least half (50–55%) of the total daily energy should come from carbohydrate. There are two different types of carbohydrate (Fig. 6.1).

Simple sugars tend to be absorbed quickly and produce a rapid increase in blood glucose levels. Complex carbohydrates are often known as slow release carbohydrates, as they take longer to be broken down into glucose. They are absorbed slowly and this leads to a more gradual increase in blood glucose levels. This means that for the patient with diabetes, the majority of carbohydrate should be in a complex form. In order to achieve the target of 50–55% of energy, complex carbohydrate foods should form the main part of the meal. Sources of refined and complex carbohydrate are given in Table 6.1.

Studies into the effects of different carbohydrate foods on blood glucose levels have shown that they can lead to different glycaemic responses (Jenkins et al 1984). This has led to the concept of the 'glycaemic index', which is defined as the glycaemic response to individual foods in relation to that of glucose.

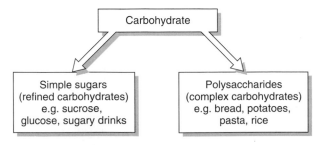

Fig. 6.1   The types of carbohydrate.

Table 6.1   Sources of carbohydrate

Refined carbohydrate (simple sugars)	Complex carbohydrate (polysaccharides)
Sweets and chocolate	Bread
Soft drinks containing sugar	Rice
Honey, jam, marmalade	Potatoes
Cakes	Cereals
Desserts	Fruit

Most studies on glycaemic index have been carried out on single foods, so the glycaemic effect of a food taken as part of a mixed meal is still not known. However it is worth encouraging patients to include low glycaemic index foods such as beans, peas, lentils, porridge and pasta as part of their diet.

Dietary fibre

This can be defined chemically as non-starch polysaccharides (NSP), which are a type of carbohydrate. Fibre is found in plant foods and it plays an important part in a healthy diet. The recommendation of 30 g per day is similar to that for the general population. There are two types (soluble and insoluble) and these are found in different foods and have different functions. Table 6.2 gives some sources.

Insoluble fibre acts like a sponge and absorbs water in the large bowel. This can help to prevent and relieve constipation and other bowel problems. It also adds bulk to the diet and can have the effect of increasing satiety by giving a feeling of 'fullness'. This can be useful in assisting weight loss. Both insoluble and soluble fibre can

Table 6.2   Sources of dietary fibre

Insoluble fibre	Soluble fibre
Wholemeal bread	Peas
Wholemeal flour	Beans
Wholewheat pasta	Lentils
Brown rice	Oats
High fibre breakfast cereal	Fruit (especially citrus)

help glycaemic control as carbohydrate foods rich in fibre take longer to digest and lead to a slower, steadier rise in blood glucose levels. Studies have shown that soluble fibre is more effective than insoluble in improving blood glucose, glycated haemoglobin and lipid levels (Fuessl et al 1987, Vinik & Jenkins 1988). Patients should therefore be encouraged to choose high fibre sources of complex carbohydrate, especially those rich in soluble fibre, e.g. pulses (peas, beans and lentils), oats and citrus fruits. Box 6.4 gives some practical tips for increasing fibre intake.

Sugars

The 1992 recommendations state that up to 25 g (1 oz) of sugar can be included as part of a healthy diet for diabetes. This may cause confusion and needs to be looked at in practical terms. The diet for diabetes is a 'low sugar' one and not 'sugar-free'. Instinct can make the newly diagnosed person with diabetes study all packets and tins for nutritional information that he/she may otherwise have ignored. Having been told to follow a 'sugar-free' diet, the patient may then avoid foods which are actually suitable as part of their diet (e.g. tinned baked beans, tinned soups and other items which contain a small amount of sugar). Emphasising that it is the very obviously sweet foods such as cakes, chocolates, sweets and sugary drinks that should be avoided will help to allay fears. In addition it should be emphasised that savoury products containing a small amount of sugar will have no effect on blood glucose when taken as part of a high fibre diet.

The allowance of 25 g (1 oz) of sugar is for use in baking, providing it is consumed as part of a high fibre, low fat diet and that it is spread

---

Box 6.4   Practical tips for increasing fibre intake

1. Aim for 5 portions of fruit and vegetables daily (including 1 oz of pulses if possible).
2. Choose wholemeal, wholegrain or granary breads.
3. Try wholegrain breakfast cereals or those based on oats, e.g. porridge.
4. Use some wholemeal flour in baking (try half wholemeal and half white).
5. Choose biscuits or crackers containing wholemeal flour.
6. Try brown rice and wholemeal pasta (or half white and half wholemeal pasta).

throughout the day. It is not recommended for those who are overweight. Sugar should only be used where its bulking and creaming properties are required (e.g. when making low sugar cakes) and artificial sweeteners should be used where possible (e.g. for drinks, milk puddings and cereals). Any sweetener based on aspartame, saccharin or acesulfame K can be used as they are all virtually calorie free and have no effect on blood glucose levels.

Fat

Fat intake should be limited due to the increased risk of arterial disease in people with diabetes. Fat should make up no more than 35% of the total daily energy intake. The main aim is to reduce the amount of saturated fat. This can be achieved by choosing alternatives to full fat dairy products, fatty meat and saturated cooking fats/ spreads. Small amounts of polyunsaturated and monounsaturated fats should be used to replace the saturated fat. Tips for reducing fat intake are given in Box 6.5.

Fat is also a concentrated source of energy, and weight for weight contains twice the energy of carbohydrate or protein.

Box 6.5 Practical tips for reducing fat intake

1. Choose lean cuts of meat and trim off any visible fat.
2. Make more use of chicken and turkey (without the skin), oil-rich fish such as herring, mackerel and kippers and white fish such as haddock, cod and lemon sole.
3. Use spreading fat sparingly. Choose one high in poly- or monounsaturates.
4. Try baking, grilling, boiling, steaming, poaching or microwaving food instead of frying.
5. Grate or slice cheese thinly and try lower fat cheeses (e.g. Edam, reduced fat cheddar and cheese spreads).
6. Choose fruit, low fat yoghurts or bread more often than biscuits, cakes and pastries if snacks are required.
7. Eat fewer fatty meat products such as sausages.

Box 6.6 Energy value of nutrients

- 1 g carbohydrate = 3.75 kcal
- 1 g protein = 4 kcal
- 1 g fat = 9 kcal

Reducing fat intake will automatically reduce energy intake, which has obvious benefits for the person who needs to lose weight. For the person whose weight is in the ideal range, an increase in complex carbohydrate will be required to make up for the deficit in calories from fat, or weight loss will result.

Protein

People with diabetes should avoid a higher than average protein intake. This is because they are more at risk of developing renal disease and a reduction in dietary protein may reduce albuminuria and glomerular filtration rate in early nephropathy (Zeller et al 1991). Between two and three servings of protein foods daily are adequate, in addition to low fat milk for use in drinks and cereal (see Box 6.7 for suggested serving sizes). Lower fat protein foods such as chicken, fish, lean red meat and pulses should be chosen in preference to higher fat meat products such as pies and sausages.

Salt

Hypertension is common in people with NIDDM and is a risk factor for coronary heart disease. Salt restriction can reduce hypertension, and the diet for diabetes should be no higher in salt than that for nondiabetics. A high intake of manufactured foods such as cheese, salty snack foods and processed meats can result in a high salt intake. Patients should be advised to use less salt in cooking (adding herbs and spices for more flavour), to taste food before salting it and to avoid adding extra salt at the table.

Alcohol

There is no need for the person with diabetes to avoid alcohol completely. The 'safe' limits for alcohol for diabetics are in line with those produced by the Health Education Authority for nondiabetics. A weekly maximum of 21 units per week for men and 14 units per week for women is advised. Box 6.8 shows how much alcohol is equivalent to one unit.

Box 6.7 Approximate serving sizes for protein foods

1 serving = 3 oz meat = 2 oz cheese = 4 oz cottage cheese = 4–5 oz fish = 4–5 oz poultry = 2 eggs

Box 6.8   Alcohol equivalents
One unit of alcohol = 1 glass wine = 1 pub measure spirits = half pint beer or lager = 1 glass sherry

Alcohol can act as a very potent hypoglycaemic agent as it inhibits the formation of glucose by the liver (gluconeogenesis). This can have very serious effects for those controlled on sulphonylureas or insulin if alcohol is consumed on an empty stomach. The advice would be to avoid drinking alcohol on an empty stomach and to eat something shortly after drinking due to the fact that the hypoglycaemic effect can last for several hours.

Diabetic products

A recent discussion paper on diabetic products (British Diabetic Association Nutrition Subcommittee 1992b) concluded that 'these products have no place in the current management of diabetes'. They were recommended in the era of the low carbohydrate diet and provided a welcome treat for those who had a taste for sweet foods. In light of the current recommendations, there is no evidence to suggest that they offer any advantages. They contain large amounts of sorbitol and fructose which can act as laxatives, they can be higher in fat than their nondiabetic equivalents and they tend to be expensive. The recommendations do allow for a small amount of sugar to be included as part of a healthy diet, which means that there is no need for 'diabetic' products. Reduced calorie or sugar-free drinks and jellies, tinned fruit in natural juice and low sugar jams and marmalades are healthier choices. These also tend to be cheaper than diabetic foods, lower in calories and available in most supermarkets.

In practical terms, the BDA dietary recommendations for the 1990s can be summarised as:

- Avoid being overweight.
- Eat regular meals.
- Make high fibre carbohydrate the main part of each meal.
- Eat less fat and exchange saturated fat for polyunsaturated and monounsaturated.
- Eat about 400 g (1 lb) fruit and vegetables daily, i.e. about 4–5 servings per day including 25 g (1 oz) of pulses, nuts or seeds.

- A small amount of sugar (25 g daily) may be included in a healthy diet.
- Special diabetic products are not necessary.
- Limit salt intake.

SPECIAL DIETARY CONSIDERATIONS FOR PATIENTS WITH NON-INSULIN-DEPENDENT DIABETES MELLITUS (NIDDM)

Overweight and obesity

75% of non-insulin-dependent diabetics are overweight, and losing weight will play a central role in their management. The only way to do this is to consume less energy than the body needs. This means that the deficit will be produced by burning body fat stores and weight loss will result.

Weight reduction can help to improve blood glucose and lipid levels as well as to reduce insulin resistance. As mentioned in Chapter 4, it has also been shown that losing weight can improve life expectancy in overweight people with NIDDM by an average of 3–4 months for each 1 kg (2.2 lb) of weigh lost (Lean et al 1990). It is therefore worth stressing the benefits of any weight loss (no matter how small) for the overweight NIDDM patient.

Assessing body weight: to manage overweight and obesity, it is important to measure and define it in terms of its relative health risk. The Body Mass Index (BMI) has been adopted widely as the best method of assessing the degree of obesity or overweight in a patient. The BMI is calculated by applying the formula:

$$BMI = \frac{Weight\ (kg)}{Height^2\ (m^2)}$$

(Weight is without shoes and in indoor clothing, and height is without shoes.) The ideal range for BMI is 20–25 kg/m^2 (Box 6.9).

Patients with diabetes should ideally have a body mass index in the 20–25 range, as both diabetes and overweight are risk factors for coronary heart disease.

Waist-hip ratio: studies suggest that the distribution of excess fat on the body is important in determining the risk of obesity

Box 6.9   Classification of obesity using BMI

- <20   = underweight
- 20–25   = 'normal'
- 25–30   = overweight/'plump'
- 30–40   = moderately obese
- >40   = severely obese

(Baumgartner et al 1987, Donohue et al 1987). Both diabetes and coronary heart disease are linked with abdominal obesity, where fatty tissue is deposited centrally giving an apple shape, rather than on the hips and thighs giving a pear shape (see also Ch. 4). Measuring the waist-hip ratio can determine where fat is deposited. A waist-hip ratio of more than 1.0 in men or more than 0.8 in women is an indicator of increased risk.

The general dietary guidelines need to be incorporated into a controlled energy intake for the overweight NIDDM patient. Dietitians work out individualised meal plans for each patient for the appropriate degree of energy restriction. Restricting the energy intake by 500 calories per day should produce a weight loss of 0.5 kg (1 lb) per week, while an energy deficit of 1000 calories per day should result in a deficit of 1 kg (2 lb) per week. In other words if a patient who usually consumes 2000 kcal per day reduces this by 500 kcal daily to 1500 kcal, he/she would expect to lose an average of 0.5 kg per week. Weight loss should be gradual, and any weight reducing programme should be based on realistic expectations of weight loss (0.5–1 kg or 1–2 lb per week is ideal). Energy intakes of less than 800 calories per day are not recommended, as they can result in loss of lean body tissue. This will affect metabolic rate and may result in less weight being lost in the long term.

Diet and oral hypoglycaemic agents

Drugs may be required if diet alone fails to control diabetes adequately, but they should not be used as an alternative to diet. Patients should be aware of the central role of diet in controlling diabetes and the overweight should be aware that losing weight will improve glycaemic control.

The mode of action of the different drugs available are discussed in more detail in Chapter 4.

Sulphonylureas

Sulphonylureas can cause an increase in appetite, leading to overeating and weight gain. This in turn can lead to a deterioration in glycaemic control. Patients should be made aware of the possible effects of these drugs and appropriate dietary counselling should be available to prevent or minimise weight gain. Although it is beneficial for everyone to eat regularly, it is especially important for those on sulphonylureas, as hypoglycaemia can result if meals are missed. For this reason, they should also be advised to avoid drinking alcohol on an empty stomach due to the combined hypoglycaemic effects of alcohol and sulphonylureas.

Biguanides (e.g. Metformin)

Biguanides do not increase appetite and are therefore usually the preferred drug for the overweight patient with NIDDM.

Glucosidase inhibitors (e.g. Acerbose)

These agents act as enzyme inhibitors and delay the breakdown and digestion of carbohydrate. This has the effect of reducing the rise in blood glucose levels after a meal. They do not cause an increase in appetite, but can cause flatulence, diarrhoea and abdominal distension.

Exercise

Regular exercise has positive benefits in that it can lower blood pressure and blood lipids. It may also reduce insulin requirements and improve overall blood glucose control. For the overweight NIDDM patient, exercise will have the added benefit of increasing energy expenditure which, when combined with a healthy diet, should assist weight loss. Regular exercise also helps to maintain lean body mass. This prevents the lowering of metabolic rate, which can be a danger with prolonged dieting.

Case Study 6.1

A 54-year-old married man has just joined the Practice. His routine medical examination shows that he has glycosuria. He is obese and consumes more than 30 units of alcohol per week. On further questioning he enjoys a fried breakfast at the weekend and takes 3 teaspoons of sugar in his tea. He admits to smoking 40 cigarettes per day and is unemployed.

On confirmation of the diagnosis, the patient will require dietary advice as his main form of treatment. There is obviously a lot of scope for improving his diet and there are many aspects to tackle. To summarise the key points:

- He is obese.
- He has a high alcohol intake.
- He may have a high fat intake.
- He has an obvious source of added sugar in his diet.
- He smokes.
- He is unemployed.

The first priority would be to explain in simple terms what diabetes is and why diet is the main element in treatment. It is important to emphasise diet and weight loss at this stage.

The advice should be broken down into stages so that he is not overwhelmed with information and the prospect of too many aspects of dietary change at once. Not all stages should be covered in the first consultation. Small, gradual changes instead of drastic ones tend to be more acceptable and lead to improved compliance.

Sugar intake

Remove sources of added sugar and foods high in concentrated carbohydrate by:

• Suggesting an artificial sweetener as an alternative to sugar. Ultimately he may be willing to take tea and coffee without any type of added sweetener.

• Assessing whether he eats sweets, sugary drinks, sweet biscuits and cakes, and advising on suitable alternatives.

Healthy eating

Emphasise that the diet for diabetes is a healthy diet:

• Advise him that this way of eating is recommended for the rest of the population and has benefits in terms of reducing the risk of heart disease.

• Encourage his wife to support him in the dietary changes and to adopt these for the family as a whole.

Smoking

Bear in mind that he is a smoker and that to stop smoking will be a very important aspect of his diabetes management. If he decides that this is his first priority, support him as follows:

- Emphasise that to prevent further weight gain would be an appropriate goal at this stage. Weight reduction can be tackled at a later stage once he has stopped smoking.
- Point out that he may find that he will lose some weight by making changes to his fat and alcohol intake.

Weight reduction

To emphasise that weight loss will help to control his diabetes:

- Explain that weight loss will only be achieved by reducing the calorie content of the diet, but that this does not mean strict 'dieting' or starvation.
- Agree a realistic target weight. Use body mass index and the patient's view of a realistic and achievable weight to aim for.
- Break down the weight loss into small goals to make the ultimate goal seem more achievable.
- Offer regular follow-up to give him support and to keep him motivated.

Alcohol intake

To encourage him to think about reducing his alcohol intake:

- Explain that his reported intake of 30 units of alcohol per week equates to at least 2400 calories.
- Negotiate a reduction in the amount of alcohol consumed.
- Advise him to avoid the special 'diabetic' beers and lagers (which have a high alcohol content) and to have ordinary beers and lagers or spirits with low calorie mixers in moderation.

Fat intake

Emphasise the importance of reducing his fat intake as follows:

- Recommend that he use alternative methods of cooking for his breakfast at the weekend (suggest grilling, baking, poaching and microwaving).
- Suggest that an ideal breakfast should contain mainly complex carbohydrate (e.g. cereal with toast), which he may be willing to consider eating on weekdays.

Financial implications

Due to the fact that he is unemployed and that cost can be a major barrier to dietary change, support him in his efforts in this way:

• Give practical advice on foods to purchase which are not more expensive (e.g. fresh fruit and vegetables that are in season and on special offer).

• Advise him of the fact that he does not require to purchase special 'diabetic' foods.

• Suggest that he makes the complex carbohydrate food the main part of his meal and has a smaller portion of the more expensive protein foods.

• Encourage him to reduce his alcohol intake and stop smoking.

Follow-up

To encourage him to make the changes:

• Offer regular follow-up so that motivation can be sustained and dietary counselling can continue.

• Reinforce the advice given by the dietitian so that information is consistent.

• Deal with each practical step at a time. Once he has omitted sugar, reduced his intake of fried food and reduced his alcohol intake, consider negotiating an increase in fruit and vegetables, wholemeal bread and wholegrain cereals. Always bear in mind that dietary change can be difficult and may be slow.

SPECIAL DIETARY CONSIDERATIONS FOR PATIENTS WITH INSULIN-DEPENDENT DIABETES MELLITUS (IDDM)

The dietary advice that should be given to a person with IDDM is basically the same as that for NIDDM, as the dietary recommendations apply to both. Eating regularly is important for both types of diabetes, but is particularly relevant for those using insulin.

Balancing food with insulin

Foods rich in complex carbohydrate are required to match the peak action of insulin, and hypoglycaemia can occur if inadequate carbohydrate is consumed. This means that regular meals and snacks should be eaten throughout the day and a usual meal pattern is breakfast, lunch and an evening meal with snacks mid-morning, mid-afternoon and at bedtime. The main aim is to eat roughly the same amount of carbohydrate at around the same time of day and to be able to adapt the diet for different circumstances.

Advice is essential so that an adequate carbohydrate intake can be achieved from day to day. Some form of accounting method is required when discussing the diet, but the practice of weighing foods is no longer necessary. There are two different ways of planning meals: carbohydrate exchanges and meal planning/household measures.

Carbohydrate exchanges

This is a system whereby the patients are taught the amount of carbohydrate in various foods and how to exchange them for other carbohydrate-containing foods if desired, in order to allow variety in the diet. In this respect it is a 'swap' system which allows for variety within the diet while at the same time maintaining a fairly consistent carbohydrate intake.

One carbohydrate exchange = Quantity of food which contains 10 g carbohydrate.

This does not mean a person can only have one exchange worth of the food, but rather that, depending on his/her usual meal plan, the patient would need to substitute an adequate amount of the food to obtain enough carbohydrate. The amount of carbohydrate needed daily is calculated according to the patient's energy requirement and distributed within an agreed meal plan suitable for that individual. A carbohydrate exchange list can give a guide to the swaps that can be made and some examples are given in Table 6.3.

Table 6.3 Examples of 10 g carbohydrate exchanges	
Food	Amount supplying 10 g carbohydrate
Wholemeal/white bread	1 small slice
Bread roll	half
Digestive biscuits	1
Apples	1
Tangerines	2
Potatoes	1 egg-sized

This system has both advantages and disadvantages. The benefits are that it can give confidence to newly diagnosed patients that they are in control and can prevent hypoglycaemia by ensuring an adequate minimum intake of carbohydrate. Often patients think in terms of exchanges immediately after diagnosis, but gradually learn to gauge their intake automatically and swap foods without thinking about grams of carbohydrate.

The drawbacks of the system are that it does not take into account the glycaemic response to a food, nor does it give an indication of protein, fat or energy content, which can draw attention away from these dietary components. The exchange system is also often thought to imply restriction of carbohydrate, which can result in higher fat foods being consumed at the expense of carbohydrate.

Meal planning and household measures

Here the patient is given ideas for 'swaps', but grams of carbohydrate are not mentioned. Advice on meal planning is given with emphasis on eating regular meals and snacks, eating a variety of foods, controlling energy intake, using appropriate cooking methods, including low glycaemic index foods, encouraging high fibre, low fat foods and eating more fruit and vegetables (particularly those containing soluble fibre).

Alcohol

As previously mentioned, alcohol is a very potent hypoglycaemic agent. Insulin and alcohol together can have a very serious effect if inadequate carbohydrate is eaten, as both will lower blood sugar levels. This must be emphasised to patients. They should avoid drinking alcohol on an empty stomach and ensure that they have extra carbohydrate to make up for the added hypoglycaemic effect of the alcohol. It is especially important to have a bedtime snack, as alcohol can continue to lower the blood sugar for several hours once drinking has stopped. Signs of hypoglycaemia can resemble signs of drunkenness, so that alcohol may mask the symptoms and go unnoticed. It is vital that diabetic identification is carried.

Exercise

Regular exercise is an important part of a healthy lifestyle, and patients with diabetes should be encouraged to be physically active.

For the insulin-dependent diabetic, exercise can affect blood glucose levels in 2 main ways:

• If control is poor and there is insufficient insulin, adrenaline will be released as a result of the exercise and will make blood sugars rise.

• If blood glucose is reasonably well controlled, there is usually an adequate supply of insulin. Here the main concern is hypoglycaemia as a result of exercise.

In order to avoid hypoglycaemia, extra carbohydrate should be taken before the activity. Alternatively the dosage of insulin can be reduced, but care needs to be taken not to reduce this too much. The amount of extra carbohydrate required will depend on the individual and the type of exercise undertaken. It can be taken as part of the last meal before exercise (e.g. an extra 20 g of complex carbohydrate as biscuits, fruit, yoghurt or nuts and raisins) or as a quick snack immediately before (e.g. 20 g of quicker-acting carbohydrate from a small bar of chocolate). Top-ups of carbohydrate may be required for endurance exercises in order to prevent hypoglycaemia during the exercise. Extra carbohydrate may also be required after exercising has stopped due to the fact that its hypoglycaemic effect can last for several hours. It is also worth remembering that everyday activities such as running for the bus or vigorous housework can also cause hypoglycaemia.

Illness

Any illness can affect diabetic control. Patients taking insulin or tablets will require to continue with these. If they are vomiting they should contact their GP, but insulin must never be stopped. The body's natural response to illness is to utilise more glucose. Insulin requirements rise and there is an increased risk of ketoacidosis. This means that insulin must be given. Carbohydrate must also be taken in some form and meals can be replaced with liquid, semi-solid or solid foods containing carbohydrate depending on the patient's appetite. As a guide, 10 g of carbohydrate should be taken every hour until they feel better. Regular blood testing is essential in times of illness. Table 6.4 gives some suggestions for carbohydrate sources during illness.

Table 6.4 Suggested carbohydrate sources during illness

Food	Amount supplying 10 g carbohydrate
Lucozade	50 ml/2 fl oz
Fruit juice	1 small glass (100 ml/4 fl oz)
Milk	1 cup (200 ml)
Thick soup	1 cup (200 ml)
Ice cream	1 briquette (1 scoop)
Yoghurt	half tub low fat/1 tub 'diet'

Case Study 6.2

A 35-year-old nurse who has IDDM works night duty every 6 weeks for 2 weeks. She asks you how she should balance her insulin and carbohydrate while on night duty.

To deal with this problem fully, the type of insulin, its duration of action and the number of insulin injections will need to be taken into consideration. She may be on a regimen of two injections daily or on a multiple injection regimen.

A regimen of two injections daily

This will usually be a mixture of quick-acting (clear) and intermediate-acting (cloudy) insulin administered 20–30 minutes before breakfast, and 20–30 minutes before the evening meal. The principles that she employs during the day will still require to be followed when she goes onto nights but her days and nights will obviously be reversed.

The key points would be:

• The nurse would need to eat regular meals and snacks.

• Accessibility of food is important (e.g. does she take sandwiches in with her or does she go to the staff canteen; are snacks available on the ward?)

• She must balance food with insulin and ensure that she eats enough carbohydrate food at each meal and snack.

• Considering her activity level—is she less active on night duty? In this case she may need less food or less insulin.

- The switch-over period from days to nights may involve an alteration in her insulin dose, which will require to be discussed with her consultant or diabetic nurse specialist, and her food intake tailored accordingly.

- She may need to test her blood glucose more regularly on the days she switches duty as this is a time of change.

A multiple injection regimen

This would usually mean that she takes one injection of long-acting insulin to give a continuous background supply (usually administered at bedtime) and quick-acting insulin would then be taken before each meal. This system allows for more flexibility with timing of meals as the injection can be delayed with less rick of hypoglycaemia. It is particularly suitable for people who work shifts, as the changeover from days to nights is simpler. It would mean that she would take an appropriate amount of insulin prior to each meal, the amount depending on the amount of food to be eaten.

CONCLUSION

Diet is the cornerstone of treatment for diabetes. Dietary advice has changed over the years in light of new scientific evidence available, and this should be communicated to the patient in practical and realistic terms. All members of the health care team should be aware of the current dietary guidelines for diabetes to ensure that consistent information is given to patients and the positive aspects of dietary change emphasised.

REFERENCES

Baumgartner R N, Roche A F, Chumlea C et al 1987 Fatness and fat patterns: associations with plasma lipids and blood pressures in adults 18–57 years of age. American Journal of Epidemiology 126:614–628

British Diabetic Association Nutrition Subcommittee 1982 Dietary recommendations for diabetics for the 1980s. Human Nutrition: Applied Nutrition 36A:378–394

British Diabetic Association Nutrition Subcommittee 1992a Dietary recommendations for people with diabetes: an update for the 1990s. Diabetic Medicine 9(2):189–202

British Diabetic Association Nutrition Subcommittee 1992b British Diabetic Association's discussion paper on the role of 'diabetic foods'. Diabetic Medicine 9:300–306

Brunzell J D, Lerner R L, Porte D, Bierman E L 1974 Effect of a fat-free high carbohydrate diet on diabetic subjects with fasting hyperglycaemia. Diabetes 23:138–142

Department of Health and Social Security Committee on Medical Aspects of Food

Policy (COMA) 1984 Diet and cardiovascular disease. Report on Health and Social Subjects 28. HMSO, London

Donohue R D, Abbott E, Bloom D M et al 1987 Central obesity and coronary heart disease in men. Lancet 1:821–824

Fuessl H S, Williams G, Adrian T E, Bloom S R 1987 Guar sprinkled on food: effect on glycaemic control, plasma lipids and gut hormones in non-insulin dependent diabetic patients. Diabetic Medicine 4:463–468

James W P T, Ferro-Luzzi A, Izaksson B, Szostak W B 1988 Healthy nutrition. WHO Regional Publications No 24. World Health Organization, Copenhagen

Jenkins D J A, Wolever T M S, Jenkins A L, Josse R G, Wong G S 1984 The glycaemic response to carbohydrate foods. Lancet 2:388–391

Lean M E J, Powrie J K, Anderson A S, Garthwaite P H 1990 Obesity, weight loss and prognosis in Type 2 diabetes. Diabetic Medicine 7:228–233

Miettinen M, Turpeinen O, Karvonen M N, Elosuo R 1977 Cholesterol-lowering diet and mortality from coronary heart disease. Lancet 2:1418–1419

Simpson R W, Mann J I, Eaton J, Carter R D, Hockaday T D R 1979 High-carbohydrate diets and insulin dependent diabetes. British Medical Journal 2:523–525

Vinik A I, Jenkins D J A 1988 Dietary fibre in the management of diabetes. Diabetes Care 11:160–173

Zeller K, Whittaker E, Sullivan L, Raskin P, Jacobson H R 1991 Effect of restricting dietary protein on the progression of renal failure in patients with insulin dependent diabetes. New England Journal of Medicine 324:78–84

Monitoring diabetes

Joan McDowell

7

INTRODUCTION

Monitoring diabetes is frequently undertaken but often without any specific thought as to why, how or when. Recent research has clearly demonstrated the link between diabetic microvascular complications and elevated blood glucose levels in patients with IDDM (The DCCT Research Group 1993). Hence the urgency to achieve normal blood glucose levels. There is probably a similar link between macrovascular complications and blood glucose levels. In addition, it is likely that these findings will be just as valid in patients with NIDDM.

Health care professionals are closely involved with monitoring diabetes. Monitoring assists in the management and evaluation of patients with the disease. Diet and therapy can be adjusted in the knowledge of home monitoring results to reach an optimum level of glycaemic control for each individual patient.

Patients taught how to monitor their own condition can be

empowered to regain control over their lives and become more responsible for their metabolic control. Self-monitoring improves the patient's understanding of their diabetes and assists the patient to maintain day-to-day control. This reduces the risks of the long-term complications of diabetes. Self-monitoring can be likened to brushing one's teeth—a little attention on a regular basis can avert a lot of future problems.

Hypoglycaemia has long been recognised as an inevitable side-effect of the sulphonylurea oral agents and insulin therapy. The DCCT research (1993) demonstrated that the achievement of near-normal glycaemia was at the expense of a two- to threefold increase in the incidence of severe hypoglycaemia. Home blood glucose monitoring (HBGM) has therefore become even more critical for the patient with tight metabolic control. Monitoring of blood glucose is necessary for the 'fine-tuning' of insulin dose (or sulphonylurea dose) and allows the patient to maintain near-normal blood glucose levels with as few episodes of hypoglycaemia as possible.

Case Study 7.1

A 56-year-old man has just been diagnosed as having non-insulin-dependent diabetes mellitus (NIDDM). He has a strong family history of NIDDM and is therefore not totally surprised at the diagnosis. He is aware of the long-term implications of the disease. His initial management is by diet alone. On questioning him, he remembers his mother testing her urine for glucose. His brother, who also has NIDDM, has just started testing his own blood glucose levels because his diabetes is going out of control, and the man asks how he ought to be monitoring his diabetes.

Assessing the patient

Before prescribing any self-monitoring techniques it is important to assess the patient in three areas.

The first is to determine how willing the patient is to perform self-monitoring. To initiate monitoring when the patient is totally unwilling to cooperate is a waste of everyone's time.

The second area to consider is whether the patient is physically able to undertake the test. Physical constraints, for example visual deficits or a lack of manual dexterity, may prevent or inhibit testing. Alternatively an inability to read either the time or results, or a lack of understanding of either spoken or written English, will make monitoring more difficult to teach and to comprehend.

The third area to consider is whether the patient will adjust the relevant therapy in the light of monitoring results. It is well documented that this is poorly done or often not done at all (Ch. 5; Leese et al 1994, Patrick et al 1993).

If monitoring is envisaged by the patient as being of value only to the health care team, then frequent clinic visits will seem essential and home monitoring results the focus of the consultation. This attitude does not promote patient empowerment.

Alternatively, patients may appear to monitor their diabetes when in fact they present fictitious results at the clinic. This may be because they wish to appear willing to cooperate. They hope to incur favour or commendation for 'doing as they are told' when in reality they are falsifying their results. Honesty and openness are essential elements in promoting empowerment.

The patient in this case study appears eager and willing to monitor his diabetes. Assuming that he has no problems in undertaking the test and reading the results, then monitoring can proceed. The challenge is to teach the patient the meaning of his results and how to alter his diet in response to them.

MONITORING OPTIONS

What monitoring options are available for this man? He may monitor either his urine or his blood for glucose. His choice of technique would depend on several factors. He should be presented with the advantages and disadvantages of both techniques, which will influence his decision. He may also decide that one particular method suits his lifestyle better than another.

Urine testing

Urine testing is the traditional way to monitor diabetes and has the advantages of being cheap, easy to use and painless to carry out. Some patients, however, find the concept of urine testing 'dirty' or unpleasant. A double-voided sample (explained below) is the best one to test; however not all patients are able or willing to comply in obtaining this sample.

Testing for glycosuria only reflects what has been happening to the blood glucose since the bladder was last emptied. Hence it only gives a relatively crude assessment of diabetic control. It gives no indication of the current blood glucose level, nor does it demonstrate fluctuations in levels. The amount of glycosuria is also influenced by the renal threshold for glucose, which is affected by many factors (Box 7.1). The renal threshold can be visualised as a dam for glucose. It is only when the blood glucose level exceeds the level of the dam that there will be any glycosuria.

The bladder acts like a reservoir and stores urine until the person urinates. Patients are advised to empty their bladders, drink a glass of water and urinate again. This second sample (called double-voided) is the one to test for glycosuria. The double-voided sample is considered more accurate than the first 'stored' sample.

Any glycosuria present roughly reflects an elevated blood glucose level. In an adult this is usually when the blood glucose is above 10 mmol/l. Therefore a mild hyperglycaemia which is below 10 mmol/l will not be reflected in glycosuria.

Likewise a negative result for glycosuria cannot be related to a particular level of blood glucose. A negative result only implies that the blood glucose has been below the renal threshold since the last time the patient passed urine. It gives no indication of impending hypoglycaemia, which may be potentially dangerous for the patient.

Those patients on sulphonylureas or insulin who show persistently negative urine results may be 'overtreated' and require to have their therapy adjusted downwards to prevent hypoglycaemia. By contrast, those patients who like to have 'a touch of sugar in the

---

Box 7.1 Factors that affect the renal threshold

- lowers during pregnancy
- lower in children and increases with age
- increases with duration of diabetes
- time of day: it varies throughout the normal day
- population groups: it varies among different populations
- medications: ascorbic acid and salicylates give a false positive result
- fluid intake and urine concentration

urine' may in fact have blood glucose levels well in excess of 10 mmol/l.

Procedure

Before proceeding to teach urine testing to the man in Case Study 7.1, an estimation of his renal threshold should be obtained. This can be done by testing a double-voided urine sample for glucose, and at approximately the same time obtaining a blood glucose result. If the two results are compatible with a renal threshold of 10 mmol/l then, should he so choose, he would be taught this method of monitoring.

The testing of urine with dipsticks is familiar to most health care professionals and is given in Boxes 7.2 and 7.3. An innovative record-

---

Box 7.2   Equipment for urine testing

- disposal gloves for the nurse
- a clean container for the sample (optional)
- urine testing dipsticks
- a watch or clock with a second hand
- diary to record results

Box 7.3   Procedure for urine testing

- The nurse wears gloves.
- The expiry date of the urine testing sticks must be checked.
- The urine to be tested should be the second sample passed at the required time and collected in a clean container.
- One urine dipstick should be removed from the container and the lid replaced securely.
- The dipstick should be briefly dipped into the urine sample and the time noted. When removing the dipstick, it should be wiped along the rim of the container to remove any excess urine.
- Alternatively, the dipstick may be passed through the stream of urine at time of voiding and the time noted.
- After the appropriate time the colour reaction is compared with the side of the container according to the manufacturer's instructions.
- Results should be recorded and brought to every clinic attendance to assist in the management of the patient.
- Store the urine testing sticks container in a safe, dry place away from children.

ing diary has been designed for those who have problems with vision, who are illiterate or lack a command of the English language (Weedon & Curry 1994).

Frequency of urine testing and its meaning

There is no consensus on the optimal frequency of urine testing. It is generally recommended that four tests are obtained each week. A pre-breakfast test reflects how well the pancreas has 'caught up' with glucose levels overnight. A test 2 hours after the main meal of the day (which may be lunch or evening meal) reflects how well the pancreas copes with a glucose load. Testing at these times twice a week gives an overall guide of diabetic control. The patient should be taught how to record these results and advised to bring this record book to every clinic attendance. The significance of the results should also be explained to the patient.

Deteriorating control would be evident first in the post-prandial test—reflecting a lack of ability to respond to a glucose load. Any persistent glycosuria in the fasting samples indicates that the blood glucose level has been elevated overnight and the patient's management should be reviewed.

Home blood glucose monitoring (HBGM)

The man in this case study may however request to test his blood glucose level, like his brother.

HBGM has the advantage of being accurate when the procedure is done properly. It reflects the blood glucose concentration at a precise time. HBGM also allows the patient to evaluate the effect of diet, exercise and lifestyle interventions on his blood glucose levels. The main disadvantages are that it is complicated to perform, and incorrect technique will produce misleading results. It is painful and some patients find it quite unacceptable.

The principles of patient assessment also apply before commencing on this education programme.

Procedure

The procedure is detailed here and in Boxes 7.4 and 7.5. The equipment required and procedure are more complex than for urine testing (Boxes 7.2, 7.3). The community nurse who is performing this procedure on patients should wear gloves to protect him/herself.

The patient's hands should be washed in warm water prior to test-

---

Box 7.4   Equipment for HBGM

- disposal gloves for the nurse
- patient's hands washed prior to the procedure
- a finger-pricking device with a measure-controlled platform
- cotton wool or paper tissues
- a watch or clock with a second hand
- blood glucose testing sticks
- disposal container for finger lancet
- meters are optional and if used, cotton wool or paper tissues may not be required
- diary to record results

Box 7.5   Procedure for HBGM

- The nurse wears gloves.
- The expiry date of the blood testing sticks must be checked.
- Patient's hands are washed in warm water. This not only cleanses the skin but also promotes blood flow to the fingertips.
- To reduce the pain the finger should be pricked on the side, using an appropriate device. Testing should be rotated around all the fingers.
- The patient should be taught how to 'milk' the finger to acquire a drop of blood.
- The drop of blood is applied to the blood glucose testing strip according to the manufacturer's instructions.
- The process is timed accurately.
- After the appropriate time the strip is wiped with cotton wool or paper tissues (depending on which blood glucose strips are used).
- A further timed period may be required before visually comparing the result with the colour chart on the side of the blood glucose strip container.
- Results should be recorded and brought to every clinic attendance to assist in the management of the patient.
- The testing sticks container should be stored in a safe, dry place away from children.

---

ing. This not only cleanses the skin but also promotes blood flow to the fingertips. To reduce the pain the finger should be pricked on the side, using an appropriate device. Testing should be rotated around all the fingers. The patient should be taught how to 'milk' the finger to acquire a drop of blood. This is then applied to the blood glucose testing strip according to the manufacturer's instructions and the process timed accurately. The strip may be wiped with cotton wool or paper tissues (depending on which blood glucose strips are used). A further timed period may be required before visually comparing the result with the colour chart on the side of the blood glucose strip container. Those patients or community nurses who have access to a blood glucose meter are encouraged to use it and follow the manufacturer's instructions regarding wiping the blood glucose strip or not. Results should be recorded and brought to every clinic attendance to assist in the management of the patient.

Learning psychomotor skills requires practice. This practice consists of repetition within a safe, non-threatening environment (Quinn 1995). To help eliminate error in this procedure, the patient should be taught how to perform HBGM, observed doing so, encouraged to practise and demonstrate the skill to the community nurse and thereafter reassessed annually. The patient may be reassessed if there is any dubiety about his results.

Fingerpricking lancets should be disposed of safely inside a firm plastic container, which should be secured before being deposited in the dustbin. In some areas, local policies have been established whereby patients deposit used lancets in the local health centre. Fingerpricking devices are freely available to patients from hospital clinics or directly from the manufacturers. Patients should not be encouraged to share fingerpricking devices with family members or friends without first changing the lancet and platform to reduce the risks of cross-infection.

Frequency of HBGM and its meaning

For patients with NIDDM, the times for HBGM should be the same as for urine testing—pre-breakfast and 2 hours after the main meal, twice a week. The results still reflect, respectively, how well the pancreas has 'caught up' with glucose levels overnight and how the pancreas responds to a glucose load.

The fasting blood glucose sample however provides the most important result since it correlates well with overall diabetic control in patients with NIDDM (Paisey et al 1980).

Urine testing or HBGM for patients with NIDDM?

While urine testing is easy to perform in comparison with HBGM, HBGM gives a more accurate picture of blood glucose levels at one particular point in time. Hence, any patient with NIDDM who requires insulin therapy would be strongly encouraged to monitor their blood glucose levels.

HBGM should also be advocated for the young, motivated patient with NIDDM, in order to protect him or her from diabetic complications and to prepare the patient should insulin therapy be required in the future.

For those patients who are almost on the maximum dose of oral agents and/or whose control is poor, HBGM should be encouraged as there is every possibility that these patients will need insulin therapy.

Those patients whose diabetes is controlled by diet alone and diet and a biguanide may opt for urine testing or HBGM. If urine testing is chosen then the patients may aim for no glycosuria without the fear of hypoglycaemia.

For the older NIDDM patient who is poorly motivated or unable to undertake the more complicated HBGM procedure, urine testing would be a reasonable option.

Many community nurses utilise urine testing frequently. Provided the community nurses have the facilities to test a blood glucose level, if they so wish, then urine testing is a rough guide to work from.

Some authors have demonstrated that for patients with NIDDM there is no significant difference in diabetic control between those patients who monitor their urinary glucose levels and those who perform HBGM (Gallichan 1994, Leese et al 1994, Patrick et al 1993). There may however be little that patients with NIDDM can do to improve control without medical advice, unlike patients with IDDM. Another study failed to demonstrate a significant difference between those who monitored their control and those who did not use any form of monitoring (Patrick et al 1993). Therefore it is possibly not important which method the patient with NIDDM actually uses for monitoring.

However, what do the patients think? One study demonstrated that most patients preferred to undertake urine testing (Gallichan 1994) and another advocated that those patients who undertake HBGM should be carefully selected for this (Leese et al 1994). This recommendation for close selection is based on the findings of the study. Patients who used HBGM showed no improvement in their diabetic control when compared with those who were urine testing. Few patients changed their own insulin in the light of their results and many of the patients would have preferred urine testing alone (Leese et al 1994).

Whichever form of monitoring a patient chooses, he/she should be supported in the choice and encouraged to take an active role in self-management. Self-monitoring should be continually reinforced, and support given to enable the necessary lifestyle changes to occur. All these aspects readily fall within the domain of the diabetic nurse specialist supported by both community and hospital nurses.

MONITORING OF PATIENTS WITH NIDDM BY THE PRIMARY HEALTH CARE TEAM (PHCT)

To acquire some objective assessment of diabetic control, a fasting blood glucose, random blood glucose or glycated haemoglobin result can be obtained.

The fasting blood glucose and random blood glucose

Most NIDDM patients retain some secretion of insulin from their beta cells. Hence a 24-hour glucose profile of the patient with NIDDM is very similar to the normal person's profile although the levels are significantly higher. A fasting blood glucose or a random blood glucose will therefore give a fairly accurate reflection of glucose levels throughout the day (Gill et al 1994, McCance & Kennedy 1991, Paisey et al 1980). As the fasting blood glucose is less likely to be influenced by what has recently been eaten, this result is probably the most important.

In a clinic setting, however, caution must be exercised in interpreting random blood glucose levels. A recent study demonstrated that a third of patients altered their diet or oral hypoglycaemic agents prior to attending a hospital clinic in attempts to achieve a lower blood glucose result (Gold et al 1994).

The stress of hospital clinic visits may have the opposite effect on blood glucose levels, causing a 'white coat hyperglycaemia' (Campbell et al 1992). It would be hoped that patients attending a clinic within the primary care setting would be less likely to demonstrate these differences. In the community, patients have a recognised relationship with their community nurse and general practitioner and so should not feel the need to alter their habits prior to a clinic. It is also hoped that patients would not feel stressed by a community clinic attendance.

The community nurse may monitor diabetes in the elderly or disabled person, in the patient's home. A planned monitoring programme can be followed whereby a random blood glucose is obtained every 4 weeks. The patient's own monitoring results can be reviewed and any other issues discussed. Through such a review, the patient may be motivated to persevere with self-monitoring and the opportunity is provided to give psychological support to the patient and carers.

The PHCT can then monitor a fasting or random blood glucose level every 3 months for an assessment of overall control for their patients with NIDDM.

Glycated haemoglobin

The term glycated haemoglobin has replaced glycosylated haemoglobin. Glycated haemoglobin comprises a series of minor haemoglobin components. Various proteins in the plasma will bind sugars, the amount of which depends on glucose levels. The higher the concentration of glucose that is present in the blood, the more will be bound to these proteins. Haemoglobin is one such protein which is present in red blood cells in large amounts. As the half-life of a red blood cell is around 6–8 weeks, so this is used as an estimate of the average blood glucose concentration over the preceding 6–8 weeks.

Many different methods are available for measuring glycated haemoglobin and each method has its own 'normal range'. Laboratories will report the glycated haemoglobin result as Haemoglobin A_1 (HbA$_1$) or Haemoglobin A_1c (HbA$_1$c)—which is a subfraction of HbA$_1$. The result is reported as a percentage of total haemoglobin. It is important that community nurses involved in interpreting these results are familiar with their local laboratory's normal range.

Since a fasting blood glucose correlates well with overall diabetic control in patients with NIDDM, it is suggested that the more expensive glycated haemoglobin is restricted to an annual test (McCance et al 1988).

Fructosamine

This is another form of assay used to measure glucose binding to proteins in the blood. It reflects the average blood glucose level over the preceding 2–3 weeks and is therefore of less value than a glycated haemoglobin for assessing long-term metabolic control. It is used in research where it may be important to document improvements in glycaemic control over short periods of time. While it is not freely available throughout the UK it is a cheap test and simple to perform. It is considered to have limited use at the moment. This is because levels fluctuate widely in diabetic patients due to variations in serum protein concentrations (McCance & Kennedy 1991).

Case Study 7.2

A 25-year-old woman has been diagnosed as having insulin-dependent diabetes mellitus (IDDM). Her management is by diet and insulin therapy. She is planning her marriage for later in the year and hopes eventually to have a family. She wants to know how best to look after her diabetes because she is worried about going blind.

Prior to presenting her with monitoring options it is important first to assess her willingness and ability to undertake self-monitoring. In discussing her monitoring options, she would be strongly advised to use HBGM as it is more accurate than urine testing. HBGM in patients with IDDM gives the information necessary to allow logical alterations in insulin doses. Urine testing does not give this information. For this woman, there are several issues to consider in promoting HBGM.

Hopefully she will enjoy a certain life expectancy, which she does not wish hindered by diabetic complications. Hence the maintenance of excellent diabetic control is essential (The DCCT Research Group 1993). She also hopes to have a family in the future, so good control prior to conception and during pregnancy is important for a healthy outcome (Lowy 1991). Using insulin therapy, this woman is at risk of hypoglycaemia. While striving for excellent diabetic control, this should not be at the price of frequent hypoglycaemic episodes. To assist her with this she would be taught the principles of insulin dose adjustment (Ch. 5) and to promote this HBGM is essential.

Assessing the patient

The patient in this case study also appears willing to monitor her diabetes. There appear to be no restrictions on her ability to undertake HBGM. Through support and education, it is anticipated that she will eventually undertake self-adjustment of her insulin.

Procedure

For HBGM, the procedure would be exactly the same as outlined above for the man with NIDDM (Boxes 7.4, 7.5). However, this woman may opt to purchase one of the blood glucose meters to ensure greater accuracy in reading her results.

Blood glucose meters

Many patients now use meters to measure their blood glucose level. Meters time the recording accurately and eliminate any doubt about the colour change on the strip. However a meter is unable to correct problems of poor technique which yield misleading results (Box 7.6). The most modern meters now operate with very small amounts of blood, which helps to eliminate the problem of an insufficient sample.

When patients purchase meters it is important that they are fully instructed in various aspects concerning the meter (Box 7.7). As each meter has different specifications, the community nurse is encouraged to familiarise him/herself with one or two to appreciate the many differences.

Box 7.6   The more common problems in HBGM technique

- dirty hands
- insufficient blood on the strip
- failure to commence timing/start the meter at the correct time

---

Box 7.7   Checklist for using a blood glucose meter

- Which test strips?
- Which technique for applying a blood sample?
- Is the test strip wiped or not?
- If the test strip is wiped—how should it be wiped?
- What maintenance is required and who will do this?
- Who to contact should there be a problem?

Meters for the visually impaired

One area of neglect is meters suitable for the visually impaired. Whatever the cause of visual impairment, these people should have the same rights and access to HBGM as sighted people. However this is often not the case as there is a great dearth of meters for the visually impaired.

Those meters which are available operate on the same principle as meters for sighted people. The difference between them is that whereas the meters for sighted people have a visual read-out of the result, the meters for the visually impaired have a visual and a spoken read-out of the result.

It should be remembered that the visually impaired may find it difficult to use blood lancets and accurately apply a drop of blood to a test strip. Such patients would be unable to use a glucose meter independently even if specifically designed for them.

Those meters which are available are up to eight times more expensive than the cheapest meter.

Frequency of HBGM and its meaning

Initially the woman in the case study would be advised to perform HBGM four times each day. The times would be prior to food and injections at breakfast, lunch, evening meal and supper. After the first week, she could probably reduce these tests to every second day. A month from diagnosis, she would be advised to undertake HBGM profiles on 2 days per week. Each hospital has its own policy regarding frequency of testing but four times a day, twice a week seems to be generally accepted. This woman, if she so wished, could opt to do HBGM once a day while varying the time each day.

While this would be the recommendation for everyday living, she would be advised to increase her testing to four times a day if she were unwell, had a period of bedrest or was experiencing frequent hypoglycaemic episodes.

By testing prior to food and insulin she determines her blood glucose level at that precise time. This information is used for insulin dose adjustment (see Ch. 5) and affords her the opportunity to evaluate the effect of aspects of her lifestyle on her blood glucose levels. Examples of such lifestyle influences would include the effects of different types of exercise, the effect of taking some cake at a special event, the effect on her blood glucose level of a heavy cold. Her goal would be to achieve near-normal glucose levels which would be accomplished as a staged process.

As mentioned previously, patients do not always adjust their therapy in the light of their monitoring results and so this woman would require continual support and guidance to make sense of her HBGM results.

MONITORING PATIENTS WITH IDDM BY THE PHCT

The blood glucose profile for patients with IDDM varies considerably throughout the day as a result of the complex interactions of diet, exercise, stress and insulin dose. There is no correlation between a single blood glucose result and overall glycaemic control. Unlike the patient with NIDDM, for the patient with IDDM a fasting or random blood glucose is of little value in assessing long-term control.

Glycated haemoglobin is therefore the most important measure of overall control and this should be obtained at every clinic visit. Patients should be informed of the meaning of this test and their results discussed with them. Patients should also be encouraged to aim for a target level of glycated haemoglobin.

The patient may attend diabetic clinics either in the hospital, the local surgery or a combination of both. The frequency of these visits partly depends on available resources. Most practitioners would prefer to see their patients every 3 months for a review appointment and annually for a complete assessment of diabetes.

More frequent attention by health care professionals may be just as effective in improving diabetic control when compared to HBGM (The DCCT Research Group 1993, Worth et al 1982). Hence frequent attendance at the diabetic clinic or review by the community nurse may be just as effective in improving diabetic control as HBGM. However there are resource implications and quality of life issues to be debated.

HBGM for the elderly on insulin

Many community nurses attend elderly patients to administer their insulin injections. These patients, whether patients with IDDM or patients with NIDDM who now require insulin, are unable to care for themselves. For such patients, the aim is to relieve the symptoms of hyperglycaemia without risk of hypoglycaemia. In other words, tight glycaemic control is contraindicated (Chs 4, 5). These patients will probably not be self-monitoring and the community nurse probably tests a urine sample daily for glycosuria. In the light of the above, should community nurses be testing the patient's blood glucose instead?

As relief of symptoms is the aim and not tight diabetic control, then there is no need to undertake the more costly, painful procedure of HBGM on a daily basis. If urine testing is persistently negative then a fasting blood glucose could be obtained to ensure that the patient's blood glucose level is not too low. A reduction of insulin dose would be indicated (Ch. 5) if 3 fasting blood glucose levels below 7 mmol/l were obtained. HBGM can easily be substituted for urine testing should the patient experience symptoms of hyperglycaemia or have an intercurrent illness.

Hence, for the elderly who are community nurse-dependent, urine testing is sufficient provided a fasting blood glucose is obtained if urine tests are persistently negative.

THE FUTURE FOR HBGM

HBGM is a valuable tool for patients who wish to monitor their own diabetes and who are at risk of hypoglycaemia. For whose who wish to undertake it, it should be encouraged. However, it should not be forced upon those who have no desire to perform HBGM. Those patients who do undertake HBGM should be audited in their technique at least annually and appropriate alterations made as necessary.

Currently research is being undertaken on shining infra-red beams through a finger tip to detect the presence of glucose. This will help to eliminate errors of technique in obtaining a blood sample and also the discomfort of pricking a finger. This is still at the experimental stage.

Continuous monitoring of blood glucose levels is another research area. An alarm system could be inbuilt to the monitor which would be triggered when the blood glucose drops below a predetermined level. This would obviously be of great benefit in the early detection and treatment of hypoglycaemia. Such a system is only theoretical at present.

The ultimate goal in research is to achieve a closed-loop system whereby the patient's blood glucose level is continuously monitored and insulin delivered at the appropriate dose from an implanted insulin pump. While this may seem unrealistic it is not totally beyond the possibilities of modern technology.

URINE TESTING FOR KETONES

While testing for glycosuria has been partly superseded by HBGM, there is still an important place for urine testing for ketones.

All patients taking sulphonylurea agents or insulin therapy should be advised to increase the frequency of their monitoring during an illness. They should also commence testing their urine for ketones 4-hourly, since these patients are at risk of developing diabetic keto-acidosis. They should seek help if ketones appear in the urine or if they do not feel better within 24 hours.

Growing children and teenagers are most prone to developing ketoacidosis due to high levels of growth hormone which antagonises the action of insulin. As in all patients with IDDM, a prompt and substantial increase in insulin dose may avert hospital admission.

Since urine ketone testing sticks are probably used infrequently, those patients detailed above need to be reminded to acquire new sticks before their old ones have gone beyond the expiry date.

OTHER FACTORS WHICH MAY INFLUENCE THE MONITORING OF DIABETES

There are some patients who are meticulous in their monitoring and insulin dose adjustment yet never achieve good diabetic control. The more they worry about it, the more good control eludes them. Such patients may have a neurotic type personality, which has been linked with poor diabetic control (Gordon et al 1993). These patients may well benefit from counselling (Ch. 3). Counselling may help the patient to focus more on their life and lifestyle rather than on their diabetes. Another strategy is to encourage these patients to relax the frequency of their monitoring and work from glycated haemoglobin results only. While these patients may be reluctant to do this, in this particular case 'what the patient does not know may not harm them'. Provided this is a short-term measure then it may reduce anxiety levels, which in turn may help to reduce glucose levels.

Patients with diabetes are encouraged to live life to the full and not to let diabetes control their life. Quality of life issues can also influence the monitoring of diabetes. A study in Norway showed that self-monitoring of diabetes was considered relatively easy to adhere to when compared with other lifestyle changes, e.g. smoking, exercise, weight and diet (Hanestad & Albrektsen 1991). This same study also showed that a higher level of quality of life was associated with greater ease of adherence to the diabetic regimen.

QUALITY ASSURANCE

It is the responsibility of the health care team to ensure that clinical measurements are as reliable and accurate as possible, as clinical decisions are made on this basis.

Quality control of blood glucose monitoring in community practice is therefore of the utmost importance. It should assess two components of testing:

- the testing skills of the personnel
- the accuracy and performance of the testing equipment.

The PHCT may consider setting their own standards for testing the skills of the personnel and determining quality control (Ch. 12).

Members of the PHCT who are involved in urine testing and blood glucose monitoring must be adequately trained in the technique and their performance regularly assessed. One way of assessing skill is by peer assessment. Asking a colleague to assess another colleague's technique according to the agreed standard will identify any areas of possible improvement.

Alternatively, solutions of known glucose concentration could be 'tested' to evaluate performance of either a meter or visual interpretation of results. This can be further validated by testing a blood sample from a patient for glucose while double checking the result obtained from the local laboratory.

Each manufacturer gives different instructions for the use of their product. Community nurses must be aware of the differences between the products and be competent in their practice.

The frequency of quality control can be determined by the PHCT but a weekly calibration and checking of meters used in practice would not seem excessive. A record should be kept of the quality control results to assist with audit of this practice (Ch. 12).

CONCLUSION

After assessment, patients are encouraged to self-monitor either their blood or urine for glucose. Blood glucose testing gives a more precise result. The frequency of monitoring is very variable but the timing depends on whether the patient has NIDDM or IDDM. The patient should be annually reassessed in monitoring technique.

Despite self-monitoring, patients do not appear to be adjusting their therapy in the light of their results. Patients require ongoing support and encouragement from all members of the health care team to build up their confidence in therapy and lifestyle adjustments.

Some patients will be dependent on others to monitor their diabetes for them. This will include those who are community nurse-dependent and those with visual, literacy or language problems. While not ideal, it may be necessary to accept less than good control from these patients.

The health care team have various tests available to them to assess diabetic control. These should be used to encourage the patient, and not used as lie-detectors!

For all diabetics, life is for living. The monitoring of diabetes, while essential, should be a part of daily routine. Health care professionals should respect those patients who choose not to monitor their own diabetes, preferring rather to 'eat, drink and be merry for tomorrow I die'!

REFERENCES

Campbell L V, Ashwell S M, Borkman M, Chisholm D J 1992 White coat hyperglycaemia: disparity between diabetes clinic and home blood glucose concentrations. British Medical Journal 305:1194–1196
The Diabetes Control and Complications Trial (DCCT) Research Group 1993 The effect of intensive treatment of diabetes on the development and progression of long-term complications in insulin-dependent diabetes mellitus. New England Journal of Medicine 329:14:977–986
Gallichan M J 1994 Self-monitoring by patients receiving oral hypoglycaemic agents: a survey and a comparative trial. Practical Diabetes 11:1:28–30
Gill G V, Hardy K J, Patrick A W, Masterton A 1994 Random blood glucose estimation in Type 2 diabetes: does it reflect overall glycaemic control? Diabetic Medicine 11:705–708
Gold A E, Charlton J, Allwinkle J, Frier B M 1994 Potential manipulation of glycaemic

control by patients with diabetes: unreliability of random blood glucose measurements. Practical Diabetes 11:4:160–161

Gordon D, Fisher S G, Wilson M, Fergus E, Paterson K R, Semple C 1993 Psychological factors and their relationship to diabetes control. Diabetic Medicine 10:530–534

Hanestad B R, Albreksten G 1991 Quality of life, perceived difficulties in adherence to a diabetes regimen, and blood glucose control. Diabetic Medicine 8:759–764

Leese G P, Jung R T, Newton R W 1994 Home glucose monitoring in patients aged over 40 years with diabetes mellitus. Practical Diabetes 11:1:32–34

Lowy C 1991 Pregnancy and diabetes mellitus. In: Pickup J C, Williams G (eds) 1991 Textbook of diabetes, Blackwell Scientific, Oxford

McCance D R, Kennedy L 1991 The concept and measurement of 'control'. In: Pickup J C, Williams G (eds) 1991 Textbook of diabetes. Blackwell Scientific, Oxford

McCance D R, Ritchie C M, Kennedy L 1988 Is HbA$_1$ measurement superfluous in NIDDM? Diabetes Care 11:6:512–515

Paisey R B, Bradshaw P, Hartog M 1980 Home blood glucose concentrations in maturity-onset diabetes. British Medical Journal 280:596–598

Patrick A W, Gill G V, MacFarlane I A, Cullen A, Power E, Wallymahmed M 1993 Home glucose monitoring in Type 2 diabetes: is it a waste of time? Diabetic Medicine 11:62–65

Quinn F M 1995 The principles and practice of nurse education, 3rd edn. Chapman and Hall, London

Weedon L, Curry M 1994 Diabetes monitoring for all? Practical Diabetes 11:1:24–26

Worth R, Home P D, Johnston D G et al 1982 Intensive attention improves glycaemic control in insulin-dependent diabetes without further advantage from home blood glucose monitoring: results of a controlled trial. British Medical Journal 285:1233–1240

The patient with diabetic complications

Derek Gordon

The management of the diabetic patient must not only include therapy for the metabolic disorder itself but must also involve careful screening for and treatment of the complications of diabetes. Diabetic complications arise mainly from the development of large vessel (macrovascular) or small vessel (microvascular) diseases. Additional effort must be put into identifying the risk factors associated with these diabetic complications. Once identified, risk can be reduced by alteration in patient lifestyle (e.g. stopping smoking) or the introduction of specific treatment (e.g. antihypertensive therapy). Only by routine screening and early intervention can the morbidity and mortality associated with diabetic complications be reduced. It should be remembered that most newly diagnosed NIDDM patients will already have risk factors and established vascular disease by the time of their diagnosis.

Insulin-dependent diabetes is also associated with a significantly increased risk of cardiovascular disease. IDDM appears to accelerate the development of vascular disease, as demonstrated by one study which showed that childhood-onset IDDM subjects had an 11-fold increase in mortality from coronary heart disease by their early 20s (Donahue & Orchard 1992).

Case Study 8.1

A 52-year-old patient attends his GP's surgery for routine review. He works as a taxi driver and takes no regular exercise. He is known to have hypertension and ischaemic heart disease, having suffered a myocardial infarct two years earlier. He is overweight, with a BMI of 28, and he has hyperlipidaemia with elevation of triglycerides and total cholesterol, discovered when screened following his heart attack. His lipid profile results 18 months previously were: Triglycerides 3.7 mmol/l, Total Cholesterol 7.9 mmol/l, HDL Cholesterol 0.6 mmol/l. He has symptoms of peripheral vascular disease with claudication after walking about 500 yards. Despite advice from his doctor he continues to eat a diet high in fat and he smokes 30 cigarettes per day. He drinks less than 10 units of alcohol per week.

His present medications are: glyceryl trinitrate spray, isosorbide mononitrate, and atenolol for his angina along with bendrofluazide for hypertension control.

At this attendance he reports to his doctor that he has noticed increasing tiredness over the past few months and more recently he has been more thirsty. His GP checks a urine sample confirming the presence of glycosuria, and a random blood glucose is measured at 18.2 mmol/l. His blood pressure is measured at 166/94 mmHg.

This patient, who has now developed diabetes, already has well-established macrovascular disease. This would include cardiovascular disease and peripheral vascular disease. He has several risk factors for macrovascular disease including obesity, hypertension, hyperlipidaemia and smoking.

MACROVASCULAR DISEASE

This term refers to the development of atherosclerotic vascular disease which results in coronary heart disease, stroke and peripheral vascular disease. These processes are, of course, not specific to diabetes but they occur at increased frequency and with increased severity in diabetic patients. This is particularly so for patients with NIDDM and is the major cause of premature mortality in this patient group (Ch. 4). Population studies in both the UK and abroad have shown that patients with diabetes carry 2–4 times the risk of dying from coronary heart disease and stroke when compared with nondiabetics (West 1971). Diabetes adversely affects both men and women.

However, diabetes appears to impart a stronger risk of coronary disease to women than to men, thus reducing or eliminating the usual female advantage in heart disease.

This patient who has developed diabetes also has hypertension and hyperlipidaemia. It is not uncommon to find obesity, hypertension and hyperlipidaemia occurring together in patients with NIDDM or impaired glucose tolerance. The finding of these disease entities grouped frequently together in the individual patient has suggested that they may be part of a more complex metabolic syndrome, the so-called Syndrome X (Reaven 1988). Whether diabetes or impaired glucose tolerance is the primary defect, or secondary to some as yet unidentified metabolic abnormality, is an area of much speculation. Similarly, it is not yet clear how the various clinical features of the syndrome relate to each other.

The management of this patient will require the identification and appropriate treatment of his risk factors for macrovascular disease.

Risk factors for macrovascular disease

Obesity

Obesity, particularly when the fat is distributed mainly to the chest and abdomen, is more common in NIDDM patients and it is now widely accepted that this pattern of fat distribution is associated with increased incidence of coronary heart disease (Kaplan 1989). This pattern of weight distribution can be assessed by measuring the girth at waist and hip level and calculating the waist-hip ratio. (This is explained more fully in Chapter 6.) Further encouragement to reduce weight will therefore be important for this patient not only because it will be necessary for the control of his diabetes but also to reduce his risk of cardiovascular disease.

Smoking

There is undisputed evidence that cessation of smoking is beneficial to nondiabetics. The Oslo Heart Study demonstrated that the incidence of myocardial infarction could be almost halved by stopping smoking (Hjermann 1981). Although there are no randomised clinical trials addressing the effect of smoking cessation on the risk of coronary heart disease in diabetics, the detrimental effects of cigarettes are evident and no-one would dispute the need to actively discourage smoking in the diabetic population.

Hypertension

Several large clinical trials have demonstrated that lowering blood pressure reduces the incidence of strokes and cardiac failure in the general population. Antihypertensive therapy also reduces the incidence of myocardial infarction but to a lesser extent. No studies of the effects of blood pressure control on cardiovascular disease in diabetes have been carried out. It is likely that high blood pressure will be equally harmful to diabetics and it would therefore be prudent to actively screen for and treat hypertension in the diabetic population. Indeed, recently published guidelines state that hypertension associated with diabetes requires intervention at lower pressures compared with hypertension in nondiabetics (see Table 8.1) (Krans et al 1995). The diagnosis of hypertension should be confirmed with three raised readings on separate occasions before treatment is started.

The patient in this study is already taking two medications, atenolol and bendrofluazide, which reduce blood pressure. The choice of anti-hypertensive agent in diabetes may be important. Bendrofluazide is a thiazide diuretic which may worsen glucose intolerance. If used at small dosage (e.g. bendrofluazide 2.5 mg) the diuretic has the same antihypertensive effect as larger doses without impairing glucose tolerance. However, thiazides even at lower doses may cause impotence. Atenolol is a beta-blocker which may similarly impair glucose tolerance and may adversely affect the lipid profile. In addition beta-blockers can mask some of the symptoms of hypoglycaemia

Table 8.1 Targets for blood pressure control in diabetes (From Krans et al 1995, p. 32)

No end organ damage		
Age (yrs)	Systolic BP (mmHg)	Diastolic BP (mmHg)
<40	140	90
>40	160	95

End organ abnormality present (i.e. proteinuria, retinopathy or cardiovascular involvement)		
Age (yrs)	Systolic BP (mmHg)	Diastolic BP (mmHg)
<40	140	90
>40	140	90

and delay recovery from hypoglycaemic episodes. For this reason they should probably not be used in the elderly patient taking oral hypoglycaemics or on insulin. Beta-blocking drugs are also contra-indicated in patients with peripheral vascular disease. As this patient has clear symptoms of peripheral vascular disease then it would seem wise to alter his medication.

Table 8.2 lists the common types of drugs used in the treatment of hypertension and specifies the advantages or disadvantages of these agents for diabetic patients.

The patient in the study should therefore have his medications altered. The bendrofluazide and atenolol should be withdrawn. A calcium antagonist such as nifedipine would be a suitable replacement for his beta-blocker since it would act as an anti-anginal and anti-hypertensive agent without causing the problems associated with atenolol. His blood pressure control is not ideal, and should it remain poorly controlled, the introduction of an ACE-inhibitor would be recommended.

Table 8.2 Antihypertensive drugs – advantages and disadvantages for people with diabetes

Drug Type	Example	Advantages	Disadvantages
Thiazide diuretic	Bendrofluazide Hydrochloro-thiazide	Well tolerated	Raises glucose, cholesterol, triglycerides May cause impotence
Beta blockers	Atenolol Metoprolol Propranolol	Used for angina and cardiac rhythm problems	Raises glucose, cholesterol, triglycerides Worsens peripheral vascular disease, Reduces symptoms of hypoglycaemia
Calcium antagonists	Amlodipine Diltiazem Nifedipine	No adverse effect on glucose or lipids Used for angina	
Ace-inhibitors	Captopril Enalapril Lisinopril Ramapril	Specific advantage in diabetic nephropathy No adverse effect on glucose or lipids	May cause renal failure in diabetics with vascular disease affecting renal arteries

Hyperlipidaemia

Hyperlipidaemia is a general term which describes disorders of the lipids in the blood. Lipids come in the form of either triglycerides or cholesterol and they are found in the blood complexed to a variety of proteins. This lipid protein complex is termed a lipoprotein. Lipoprotein complexes come in a range of sizes and contain differing amounts of triglyceride, cholesterol and protein. Increased blood concentrations of cholesterol in the form of a low density lipoprotein complex (LDL-chol) are associated with an increased risk of cardiovascular disease. By contrast, raised levels of cholesterol in the form of high density lipoprotein (HDL-chol) are cardioprotective. Elevated triglyceride concentrations are also thought to be associated with an increased risk of cardiovascular disease. The most prevalent lipid abnormalities in diabetes are mildly elevated triglycerides or a combined increase in both cholesterol (total cholesterol and LDL-cholesterol fraction) and triglycerides.

Community nurses may be quite familiar with sending blood samples to the biochemistry laboratory requesting 'fasting lipids'. Different laboratories may report different aspects of the lipid profile including total triglycerides, total cholesterol and perhaps cholesterol subfractions such as HDL-cholesterol and LDL-cholesterol. If abnormalities in lipids are found it is important to exclude any underlying conditions which may be contributing to the hyperlipidaemia. Alcohol excess, abnormal liver function and hypothyroidism, as well as diabetes, can cause a rise in lipid levels and should be screened for.

What is the significance of these results to the care of the diabetic patient? Macrovascular disease occurs at increased frequency and at a younger age in diabetic patients and the protective advantage of the female hormones is lost. Treatment to reduce plasma lipids in the general population has been shown to reduce the incidence of angina, myocardial infarction and the need for coronary artery surgery (Frick, Elo, Heinonen et al 1987). It is likely therefore that similar lipid lowering treatments will be equally effective in reducing the incidence of cardiovascular disease in diabetic patients. There are however no clinical trials to prove this and the treatment of hyperlipidaemia in diabetes remains controversial.

Despite the controversy it would seem reasonable to screen the diabetic population for hyperlipidaemia. Total cholesterol, HDL-cholesterol and triglycerides should be measured in the non-fasting state initially and repeated in the fasting state if abnormalities are identified. It is best not to take these measurements at the time of diagnosis since initial poor diabetic control will influence the triglyceride measurements in particular. Lipids should therefore be checked once the diabetes has been treated and controlled and the measurements thereafter repeated annually.

The patient in the study is known to have raised triglyceride and cholesterol concentrations, a pattern of lipid abnormality found commonly in NIDDM patients. Hypertriglyceridaemia should be managed initially by achieving tight diabetic control, and this will involve dietary measures. Diet is fundamental to the management of lipid abnormalities in diabetics. The patient should therefore be given additional dietary advice and recommended a diet low in fat. In particular the amount of saturated fats should be restricted and the total cholesterol intake also reduced. For further information on the dietary management of diabetes and hyperlipidaemia, see Chapter 6. Target levels for blood lipids are shown in Box 8.1. Failure of diet to control hyperlipidaemia after 6 months indicates that drug treatment is necessary.

Five different classes of lipid lowering drugs are currently available. These include bile acid binding resins, nicotinic acid, fibrates, HGM CoA reductase inhibitors (statins) and probucol. Use of these drugs in the diabetic patient poses certain problems and an optimum drug regimen has not yet been defined. Table 8.3 illustrates the advantages and disadvantages of each agent.

Fibrates are probably the drug of first choice in most diabetics since they act to reduce both cholesterol and triglycerides. If high triglycerides persist, nicotinic acid analogues should be considered. If both cholesterol and triglycerides remain elevated, a fibrate should be considered plus a bile acid sequestrant or a statin with nicotinic acid analogue as additional therapy. Until recently the combination

Box 8.1 Targets for plasma lipid levels	
Patients with known vascular disease:	Total cholesterol <5.2 mmol/l Triglycerides <2.3 mmol/l
Other diabetic patients	Total cholesterol <6.5 mmol/l Triglycerides <4.5 mmol/l

Table 8.3   Lipid lowering drugs used in diabetics

Drug Type	Example	Advantages	Disadvantages
Fibrates	Bezafibrate Gemfibrozil Ciprofibrate	Lowers both cholesterol and triglycerides	
Bile acid binding resins	Cholestyramine Colestipol		Raise triglycerides Unpalatable
Nicotinic acid		Lowers both cholesterol and triglycerides	Worsens glucose tolerance
HMG CoA reductase inhibitors	Pravastatin Simvastatin Fluvastatin		Lowers cholesterol only
Probucol			Lowers cholesterol only. Must be stopped 6 months before planned pregnancy

of a fibrate with a statin was considered dangerous as both drugs can cause muscle damage (rhabdomyolysis). However the combination of bezafibrate with a statin is being used more frequently in patients with severe hyperlipidaemias.

Lack of exercise

Regular exercise will also help this patient to achieve weight loss. This has been shown to improve lipid profiles, in particular a decrease in serum triglyceride concentrations. Patients with diabetes should undertake regular exercise programmes only after they have been screened for diabetic complications. Those with cardiovascular disease, proliferative retinopathy or neuropathy affecting the lower limbs or autonomic system should exercise with caution and avoid vigorous training.

Excess alcohol intake

If alcohol consumption is greater than the recommended intake it should be reduced. The recommended maximum weekly intake of alcohol is 21 units for men and 14 units for women (Ch. 6). Excessive alcohol intake is associated with both hyperlipidaemia and hypertension. This man however admits to taking less than 10 units per week. While this is within the recommended weekly intake he should probably be advised to reduce this because of the calorie content of alcohol.

Secondary prevention

There is limited information on the benefits of secondary prevention in diabetics; that is treatment to prevent further acute events after a stroke or myocardial infarction. Nevertheless, it would seem sensible to prescribe aspirin for this patient following his myocardial infarction. Aspirin should also be given following cerebral infarction and for the treatment of transient ischaemic attacks. Similarly the benefits of beta-blockers as secondary prevention following myocardial infarction probably outweigh the disadvantages in diabetics.

Peripheral vascular disease

The patient in this case study has symptoms of peripheral vascular disease with claudication after walking about 500 yards. His GP would assess his peripheral circulation by palpating for leg pulses and listening over the femoral arteries for a bruit.

Peripheral vascular disease in diabetic patients develops more rapidly and tends to be more diffuse than in nondiabetics. The atherosclerotic process affects the arteries below the knees to a much greater extent in patients with diabetes. At the time of diagnosis of NIDDM nearly 10% of patients will already have lower extremity arterial disease. With advancing age the incidence of lower extremity disease may reach 45% after 20 years' duration of diabetes (Orchard & Strandness 1993). The presenting symptom is usually intermittent claudication affecting buttock, thigh or calf muscles. With diffuse disease affecting the extremities, claudication can also affect the muscles of the foot. With worsening peripheral circulation, pain begins to develop at rest. Rest pain typically worsens at night and may be relieved by removing the bedclothes and 'dangling' the feet over the side of the bed.

Treatment

The patient should again be encouraged to reduce weight, undertake regular moderate exercise and stop smoking. Hypertension and hyperlipidaemia have already been identified and treated. Beta-blocking drugs are contraindicated and the patient's atenolol therapy has been withdrawn. When intermittent claudication begins to restrict quality of life or rest pain develops, he should be referred to a vascular surgeon.

Screening

Screening for peripheral vascular disease is essential at initial diagnosis of diabetes and annually thereafter. This involves a careful history taking and palpation of the distal pulses. This patient is at increased risk of foot pathology and should be given appropriate advice on foot care. For further information on the management of the diabetic foot the reader is referred to Chapter 9.

Case Study 8.2

A 42-year-old married man with IDDM moves into the General Practice catchment area and applies to join the practice. He wishes to see his GP because he has developed tingling and numbness of both feet. He complains of a burning discomfort in his legs. This is worse during the night and prevents him from sleeping.

He has had diabetes for almost 20 years and is on a twice-daily regimen of a fixed mixture insulin (soluble and isophane). He claims that his diabetes is satisfactorily controlled and he never has any problems with hypoglycaemic episodes. However it is evident that he rarely monitors his own blood glucose levels and he has not attended a hospital diabetic clinic for more than 8 years. His previous GP did not run a diabetic clinic and he has not received any diabetic care over this period of time.

His GP finds on routine urine testing that there is 1% glycosuria and significant proteinuria. His blood glucose is measured at 18.2 mmol/l and poor metabolic control is confirmed by the finding of an elevated glycated haemoglobin.

There is reduced sensation to both light touch and pin-prick testing to mid-calf level in both legs. His blood pressure is noted to be elevated at 165/95 mmHg. His GP also finds changes on fundal examination of diabetic retinopathy. The GP also suspects that the patient may have developed diabetic nephropathy and measures his urea and creatinine, which are both found to be elevated at 15.8 mmol/l and 270 micromol/l respectively.

This patient with longstanding IDDM has now developed some of the complications of diabetes. These are hypertension, retinopathy, nephropathy and neuropathy.

MICROVASCULAR COMPLICATIONS

Microvascular disease affects the small blood vessels and is specific to diabetic patients. The actual mechanisms which result in damage to the small vessels are poorly understood, and detailed debate on the possible causes of microvascular disease will not be introduced here. Microvascular disease is primarily involved in the development of diabetic retinopathy and nephropathy and may also be important in the aetiology of neuropathy. In addition small vessel disease may cause diffuse cerebrovascular disease with resulting cerebral atrophy. Microangiopathy involving the small vessels of the myocardium may be responsible for the poorer prognosis in diabetic patients following myocardial infarction, and may contribute to me higher incidence of cardiac failure in such patients.

Retinopathy

Clearly prevention of retinopathy is the prime aim and tight diabetic control is the only effective means of achieving this.

Diabetic retinopathy is primarily a disease of the retinal capillaries. This later extends to the larger vessels: veins, arterioles and small arteries. The cause of the microvascular disease is poorly understood. Whatever the underlying mechanism, the results of small vessel damage are twofold:

- capillary occlusion and retinal ischaemia
- leakage from the capillaries causing exudation and oedema.

Diabetic retinopathy is graded into four main categories depending upon the extent of the disease as seen on fundal examination.

Background retinopathy

As capillaries close, the retina becomes under-perfused with blood. Surrounding capillaries dilate in response to this and microaneurisms form. These tiny, pinhead, red dots are the first lesions to be seen in developing retinopathy.

Dilated capillaries are usually leaky and proteinaceous material escapes forming creamy-white exudates (hard exudates) on the retinal surface. Large blot haemorrhages tend to form at the interface of the well-perfused and ischaemic areas of the retina (Fig. 8.1).

Advanced background retinopathy

If extensive leakage from capillaries occurs around the macula,

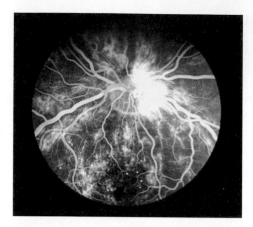

Fig. 8.1 Fluorescein angiogram of the retina. Fluorescein dye is seen escaping from the blood vessels and entering the retina. Microaneurisms are clearly seen as small rounded opacities.

macular oedema develops. Since the macula is involved with central vision, oedema of this area can markedly impair vision. The patient will usually complain of blurring of the vision, particularly his central vision which is used when reading.

As more and more capillaries become occluded, large areas of the retina become ischaemic and cotton wool spots (or soft exudates) develop at sites of retinal micro-infarction. The veins of the retina also begin to dilate. The veins form loops or show beading and reduplication. The presence of cotton wool spots and venous changes suggests that new vessel formation is imminent. Approximately one third of patients will develop new blood vessel formation within the next two years, and progress to proliferative retinopathy. Patients with advanced background retinopathy should therefore be referred to an ophthalmology clinic.

Proliferative retinopathy

Ischaemic areas of retina subsequently give rise to new blood-vessel formation. These new vessels usually arise from veins in the retinal periphery or on the optic disc. At first they lie on the surface of the retina but eventually they grow forwards, attaching themselves to the posterior surface of the vitreous which lies immediately in front of the retinal surface. As the vitreous detaches it pulls on the new vessels causing them to rupture and haemorrhage. Haemorrhaging into the vitreous causes sudden loss of vision as the blood prevents light reaching the retina behind. Vitreous haemorrhages usually clear gradually over a period of days or weeks with vision slowly recovering. Such patients require urgent referral to an ophthalmologist.

Advanced diabetic retinopathy

Repeated vitreous haemorrhages stimulate fibrous tissue proliferation. Fibrous strands arising in relation to new vessels begin to contract and as this process gradually progresses, the retina becomes detached with resulting loss of vision.

Epidemiology

Diabetic retinopathy is the commonest cause of blindness in people under the age of 65 years living in the developed world. Up to 38% of patients with NIDDM may have microaneurisms at the time of diagnosis, indicating the delay in diagnosis of these patients. In patients with IDDM it is unusual to see retinal lesions before 5 years' duration of diabetes and proliferative retinopathy is unusual during the first 10 years. Its incidence thereafter rises sharply and remains steady.

Diabetic retinopathy, especially its proliferative manifestations, is more common in patients with poor control of diabetes (Klein et al 1987). The DCCT study (DCCT Research Group 1993) has clearly demonstrated that improved diabetic control delays not only the development of retinopathy but also the progression of established retinopathy in IDDM patients (Ch. 5).

Treatment

Once macular oedema or proliferative changes have developed, the only treatment available is photocoagulation. Laser photocoagulation is particularly effective in preventing visual loss due to new vessel formation. For laser phototherapy to be effective it must be given early and be sufficiently aggressive. In 90% of patients the new vessels disappear or become insignificant. Once treatment has been successful, good vision is maintained (Sullivan et al 1990). In maculopathy, treatment is less effective with only 60% of patients achieving initial benefit (Davies et al 1989). Macular oedema responds well to photocoagulation but ischaemia of the macular area is rarely helped by laser treatment.

Laser photocoagulation is not without side-effects. The process causes retinal damage and if extensive treatment has been necessary, some visual field loss is inevitable. Colour vision is often impaired when laser photocoagulation is close to the macula.

Vitrectomy, an operation to remove the vitreous humour and surrounding fibrous tissues, is sometimes capable of restoring vision to patients blinded by advanced retinopathy.

Screening

Prevention of diabetic blindness is possible in most cases as long as treatment is initiated early. Since the initial features of retinopathy are symptomless, screening is worthwhile and cost-effective (Foulds et al 1983). The St Vincent Declaration aims to reduce the incidence of diabetic blindness by a third (Ch. 11). In order to achieve this goal, screening programmes are essential.

Impaired vision is an early feature of maculopathy and may develop before any retinal changes are evident on ophthalmoscopic examination. A falling visual acuity may therefore be the first sign of serious maculopathy developing. By contrast, patients with proliferative retinopathy will be unaware of any eye problem until a vitreous haemorrhage causes a sudden loss of vision. By this stage retinopathy will be advanced and difficult to treat effectively. It is evident therefore that any screening programme must include both the routine measurement of visual acuity and fundoscopy.

Visual acuity

Distance vision is measured with a well illuminated Snellen chart at 6 metres. Each eye is tested separately while the other eye is covered with a card. Visual acuity is quoted as the smallest letters which can be read. Thus if a patient can only read at 6 m letters which should normally be read at 24 m, visual acuity is recorded as 6/24. Normal vision is 6/6 but those with long sight and the young can often manage 6/5 or 6/4. On the other hand, vision deteriorates with age and 6/9 vision is not necessarily abnormal in the elderly. If no letters can be read, the ability to count fingers (CF), identify hand movements (HM), or perceive light (PL) should be tested and recorded. Vision should be tested with the patient wearing glasses if normally used for distance. If vision is impaired, the test should be repeated viewing the chart through a hole punched in a card (a pinhole). This partially corrects refractive errors. The best acuity measurement for each eye should be recorded.

Tests of reading ability using cards with varying sizes of script test central vision and are therefore particularly sensitive to macular changes.

Fundal examination

Fundoscopy should be carried out only by doctors with training and experience of looking at the eyes of patients with diabetes. For this reason most GPs still prefer to send their patients to a diabetic or ophthalmology clinic for retinal screening. In some areas of the country local opticians have been trained in assessing diabetic fundi and are used in screening programmes.

In order to obtain full and clear views of the retina it is necessary for the pupils to be dilated by using mydriatic drops. Tropicamide (0.5 or 1%) is the most suitable agent since it acts rapidly and wears off within 6 hours. There is little to be gained from reversing the drops using pilocarpine after the consultation. Drops are usually instilled by nursing staff, who should first check that the patient does not suffer from glaucoma. The patient should be advised previously that an eye examination will happen and warned that his vision may remain blurred for up to 6 hours after the examination. He may not wish to drive during this time.

The examination should take place in a suitably darkened room using an ophthalmoscope with a fully charged battery providing adequate illumination.

In some areas of the country non-mydriatic retinal cameras are used in screening programmes. In order for high quality pictures to be produced an experienced operator is required for the camera. Even so, new vessels at the edge of the fundus can be missed. An advantage of this technique however is that a permanent record is made of the patient's fundus for future reference and comparison.

Cataracts

Cataracts are common in diabetic patients and in general occur about 10 years earlier than in nondiabetics. Treatment of cataract is by surgical removal of the lens and replacement with an artificial plastic lens implant.

Blind registration

Blind registration can only be undertaken by a consultant ophthalmologist. The patient can be registered as either 'partially sighted' or 'blind'. The impact of blindness on an individual cannot be over-emphasized and every effort should be made to support the patient both physically and emotionally. The social services may be required to organise home support and the patient should be encouraged to remain as independent as possible. Guide-dogs may be important in this respect. Being registered blind entitles the patient to certain financial and other benefits: an increased income tax allowance, free radio and loan of talking books, etc. In addition many social services provide retraining programmes and tuition in Braille.

Nephropathy

Diabetic nephropathy rarely develops before 10 years' duration of diabetes. Those patients who go on to develop nephropathy will tend to do so over the next 20 years and those patients who survive 35 years of diabetes without developing nephropathy are at extremely low risk of doing so in the future. Altogether between 30 and 40% of patients with IDDM develop diabetic nephropathy (Fig. 8.2).

The patient in the study has had IDDM for 20 years and so it is not unusual that his GP suspected and discovered raised levels of urea and creatinine. The identification of renal impairment in a diabetic patient has serious implications. Such patients are 100 times more likely to die when compared to a nondiabetic population. IDDM patients without nephropathy only have a twofold increase in their relative mortality.

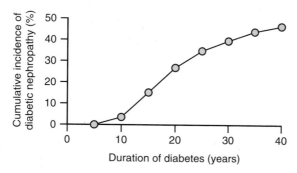

Fig. 8.2   The cumulative incidence of diabetic nephropathy in relation to duration of diabetes. (Reproduced by kind permission from Andersen A R, Christiansen J S, Andersen J K, Kreiner S, Deckert T 1983 Diabetic nephropathy in Type 1 (insulin-dependent) diabetes: an epidemiological study. Diabetologia 25:496–501. © Springer Verlag)

One of the earliest features of developing nephropathy is the presence of protein in the urine. Initially protein is present only intermittently in the urine and in small amounts. Normal albumin excretion in the urine is less than 30 mg/24 hours. However routine urine testing with dipsticks will detect proteinuria only if the albumin excretion is greater than 300 mg/24 hours. More sensitive methods have therefore been developed to measure the very small amounts of albumin (microalbuminuria) present in the urine of patients with very early nephropathy. Microalbuminuria is defined as an albumin excretion rate of 20–200 µg/min or 30 to 300 mg/24 hours. A single elevated microalbuminuria estimation is insufficient and must be confirmed by three elevated collections over a 6-month period. An albumin excretion rate can be determined most easily from an early morning urine sample. Alternatively a 24 hour urine sample can be obtained. Accuracy of complete 24 hour collections can however be a problem in clinical practice.

The presence of microalbuminuria with IDDM is highly predictive of progression to clinical diabetic nephropathy during the next 10–15 years (Mogensen & Schmitz 1988, Parving et al 1982, Viberti et al 1982).

Once routine urine testing with a dipstick becomes persistently positive for proteinuria, renal function begins to decline, with 50% of patients reaching end stage renal failure within 7 to 10 years (Andersen et al 1983, Krolewski et al 1985).

The DCCT Study has clearly demonstrated that adequate glycaemic control is required to prevent the development or progression of diabetic nephropathy. The presence of microalbuminuria should alert those health care professionals who are monitoring the diabetic patient to the need for improved metabolic control (DCCT Research Group 1993).

Many studies have shown that reducing blood pressure in patients with nephropathy slows the rate of declining renal function (Mogensen 1982, Parving et al 1987). There is some evidence that angiotensin-converting enzyme inhibitors may be particularly beneficial (Bjorck et al 1992). Recent work has suggested that ACE-inhibitor treatment may even be of benefit in patients with IDDM who have microalbuminuria but who are not hypertensive. ACE-inhibitor therapy has been shown to impede the progression to clinical proteinuria in these patients (Viberti et al 1994).

Dietary restriction of protein has also been shown to slow the progression to chronic renal failure in patients with nephropathy (Zeller et al 1991).

The patient in this case study should therefore be referred to the local hospital diabetic clinic where he will be encouraged to monitor his diabetes more carefully and given further advice regarding insulin dose adjustment. His blood pressure will be carefully monitored and treatment with ACE-inhibitor started if indicated. His renal function will be assessed and followed closely. As function deteriorates he will be referred to the nearest renal unit.

Nephropathy in NIDDM

Studies of nephropathy in patients with NIDDM are complicated by the fact that proteinuria in the elderly may be caused by other medical problems such as congestive heart failure, hypertension, vascular disease or urinary tract infection.

The incidence of proteinuria in NIDDM has been evaluated in relatively few studies, partly because it is usually difficult to know the duration of the diabetes accurately. One study estimates that about one quarter of NIDDM patients will have proteinuria after 20 years of diabetes (Ballard et al 1988). Microalbuminuria is therefore common in elderly patients with NIDDM and is predictive of subsequent clinical nephropathy and also death. However, the predominant cause of death in NIDDM patients with microalbuminuria is cardiovascular disease and not renal failure.

There have been very few studies of intervention in NIDDM patients with nephropathy. It is likely that treatment of hypertension in this group will be important in slowing the progression of the disease. There are no studies however to show that improved glycaemic control in patients with NIDDM will alter the prognosis associated with proteinuria.

Neuropathy

Diabetic neuropathies can be classified as either mononeuropathies or polyneuropathies. Mononeuropathies affect single peripheral nerves involving sensory, motor or both functions of the nerve. Polyneuropathies are mainly sensory in type and result in paraesthesia and numbness which develops in a 'glove and stocking' distribution. Neuropathy associated with diabetes is common although estimates of its prevalence vary widely depending upon the methods used to diagnose and detect the neuropathy.

The patient in the case study has developed a symmetrical poly-neuropathy. This is by far the most common diabetic neuropathy. A recent study in the UK found evidence of peripheral neuropathy in almost a third of patients attending a hospital diabetic clinic (Young et al 1993). Its prevalence increases with both age and duration of diabetes, and it is present in more than half of all patients with NIDDM over the age of 60 years.

This type of neuropathy is always bilateral and first affects the distal aspects of the lower limbs. Its sensory symptoms include burning, itching, pins and needles, cramps and tightness. These are particularly prominent during the night and patients frequently report being unable to tolerate sheets or blankets over their legs. Affected patients may also experience reduced or complete loss of sensation for all modalities: touch, pain, temperature and proprioception. When the sensory disturbance becomes severe, the loss of proprioception results in an ataxic gait, and the loss of other sensations predisposes the foot to trauma and injury with subsequent skin ulceration and joint deformity developing.

Mononeuropathies can affect individual cranial or peripheral nerves. The commonest diabetic mononeuropathy involves the third cranial nerve. A third cranial nerve palsy causes downward and lateral deviation of the eye. This is associated with a complete ptosis. Onset is usually sudden and sometimes accompanied by pain. Improvement gradually occurs over a period of months.

Single peripheral nerves may also be affected by diabetes. Common examples would be median nerve damage causing a carpal tunnel syndrome, or involvement of the ulnar nerve causing wrist drop or the peroneal nerve causing foot drop.

Diabetic amyotrophy

Diabetic amyotrophy typically presents in the patient over 50 years of age. The patient finds walking and rising from the sitting position increasingly difficult due to weakness of the proximal leg muscles. The muscles usually involved are the quadriceps, iliopsoas and thigh adductors. Examination often reveals marked wasting of the muscles of the thigh and buttocks and absent knee jerks. A deep aching pain in the affected muscles is not uncommon and often prevents sleep.

The onset of symptoms can be either acute (over a period of days) or subacute (over a period of weeks).

This syndrome is now thought to be due to neuropathy affecting the proximal peripheral nerves of the lower limbs (Chokroverty 1982, Williams & Mayer 1976).

Most patients will experience gradual recovery of muscle strength and relief of pain over a period of 1–2 years. This may involve lengthy in-patient treatment for rigorous tightening of diabetic control and for physiotherapy. Unfortunately a small number of patients experience no recovery of power and becomes severely disabled.

Treatment of neuropathy

The DCCT study has clearly demonstrated that maintenance of tight diabetic control in patients with IDDM may reduce the risk of developing neuropathy by 60% when compared with less well controlled patients (Ch. 5). Improving diabetic control also results in improved nerve function but is unlikely to reverse all the symptoms of a fully developed neuropathy. There is every likelihood that similar results can be achieved by tight metabolic control in patients with NIDDM.

The patient in the study has troublesome neuropathic pain. He should firstly be encouraged to tighten his diabetic control. He may require re-education in blood glucose monitoring and alteration of insulin dosage.

Few drugs used to treat painful neuropathy have proved effective. The tricyclic antidepressants imipramine and amitriptyline have been shown to be of benefit (Fields 1990, Kvinesdal et al 1984). However, treatment is often compromised by side-effects causing sedation, urinary retention or postural hypotension. Anticonvulsants such as phenytoin and carbamazepine have also been tried with variable results.

Autonomic neuropathy

Diabetes can frequently affect the autonomic nervous system which is responsible for the regulation of many body functions, including:

- the control of heart rate and blood pressure
- the motility of the gastrointestinal tract
- function of the genitourinary tract
- sudomotor function (sweating).

In clinical practice , the most common symptoms which are caused by autonomic neuropathy are postural hypotension, severe nocturnal diarrhoea and impotence. Lack of sweat production may not be noticed by the patient but nevertheless can cause problems when the skin of the feet becomes dry resulting in fissuring and infection. Severe and intractable vomiting can occur in patients with autonomic dysfunction affecting gastric motility and emptying of the stomach.

Patients presenting with any of these symptoms should be referred to the local diabetic consultant for further investigation and·management. Symptoms of autonomic neuropathy are difficult and complicated to treat and the long-term prognosis for these patients is poor.

Impotence

Impotence is a common problem, affecting between one third and one half of all male diabetic patients (Fairburn et al 1982). Erectile impotence is age-related and reduced potency occurs in 70–80% of all males, whether diabetic or not, by the time they reach 80 years of age. Diabetes, however, results in impotence at much younger ages in diabetic men. Once impotence has developed in the diabetic it is progressive and permanent.

Impotence is probably the most under-diagnosed complication of diabetes. This is due to the reticence of both patient and doctor to discuss sexual problems. Health care workers should therefore always be alert to the possibility of this diabetic complication and be prepared to introduce the subject into a routine consultation. This oft-unspoken complication may be causing much distress and disharmony for the patient and his partner. A sympathetic manner assists in identifying the problem. An explanation of the facts may initially reassure them both that this is a common complication of diabetes.

Several factors, both physical and emotional, may be contributing to the development of impotence. In assessing the impotent male it is important to establish that there are not any treatable causes. In this respect it is necessary to establish that there is no underlying psychological or marital problem that may have precipitated the difficulty. Impotence may itself generate psychological problems and it is sometimes difficult to determine which came first, the impotence or the emotional difficulties.

Medications and drugs may be responsible for erectile failure and a list of common drugs which cause impotence is provided (Box 8.2).

Box 8.2 Drugs associated with impotence		
Antihypertensives:	CNS depressants:	Other drugs:
beta-blockers	phenothiazines	cimetidine
bendrofluazide	haloperidol	metoclopramide
spironolactone	tricyclic antidepressants	alcohol
methyldopa		marijuana

Liver and renal function should be assessed because chronic illness and excessive alcohol consumption can predispose the male to impotence. The patient should be screened for gonadal failure and hyperprolactinaemia. However, in the vast majority of impotent diabetic patients, no significant hormonal abnormalities will be detected.

Impotence in the diabetic is due mainly to two mechanisms: vascular disease and autonomic neuropathy. Vasculogenic impotence is frequent in patients with arterial disease elsewhere, particularly peripheral vascular disease of the lower limbs. Erection requires a sixfold increase in arterial blood flow through the penis and clearly will be impaired by any impediment to this flow. The parasympathetic nervous system controls this blood flow, and autonomic neuropathy affecting the innervation of the penis will also result in erectile failure.

There are two main treatments available for impotence: vacuum tumescence or intracorporeal injection of vasoactive drugs. Vacuum tumescence devices induce erection by creating a vacuum in a solid condom apparatus which surrounds the penis. A rubber band is slipped over the cylinder and around the base of the penis to maintain the erection and the cylinder is removed (Fig. 8.3). These devices are usually supplied with explanatory videos which can be given to the patient to view in his own home. This provides the patient and partner with privacy and time to decide whether the apparatus is acceptable. With these devices most patients are able to achieve erections which allow penetration. Adverse reactions are uncommon. Bruising around the base of the penis can occur and this form of treatment is therefore not appropriate for patients with a bleeding diathesis or on anticoagulant treatment. This form of therapy could be provided in a general practice setting without the need for specialist referral.

Patients can be instructed in the self-injection of vasoactive agents

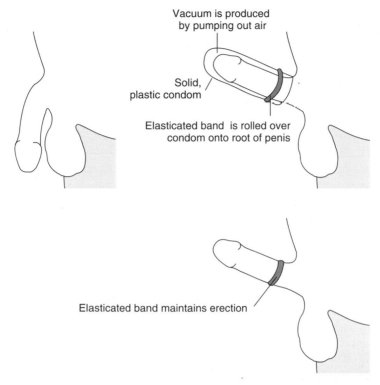

Vacuum is produced
by pumping out air

Solid,
plastic condom

Elasticated band is rolled over
condom onto root of penis

Elasticated band maintains erection

Fig. 8.3   The vacuum tumescence device for the treatment of impotence.

such as papaverine or prostaglandin E1. Injection into the corpus cavernosum of the penis requires initial supervision. A test dose is given and the dose increased gradually at following hospital visits until an adequate erection is obtained. Intracorporeal injections can cause priapism requiring hospital specialist intervention and most clinics provide contact numbers for patients in case of such an emergency. This form of therapy is therefore normally provided by a diabetologist or urologist with a special interest in such treatment.

Patients who have psychological problems related to their impotence should be referred for sexual advice. This may be available from the local RELATE counsellors, family planning clinics or, if appropriate, psychosexual counsellors.

Hypoglycaemia

Hypoglycaemia occurs commonly in patients receiving insulin therapy and occurs less frequently in patients on sulphonylurea treatment. The precise incidence of hypoglycaemia in both groups of patients is unknown and almost certainly underestimated and under-reported by patients. Patients with NIDDM who are taking sulphonylureas may fail to recognise the symptoms of hypoglycaemia, attributing sweating, palpitations, dizziness or other symptoms simply to 'old age'. Insulin-dependent patients often fail to report mild symptoms of hypoglycaemia (e.g. feeling hungry) believing that this is a 'normal' feature of being diabetic. More severe hypoglycaemia can cause retrograde amnesia or emotional denial. Thus patients may report no problems with hypoglycaemia while their partner may reveal a start-lingly different picture.

Case Study 8.3

The wife of a 60-year-old bank manager attends her GP to express concern about her husband, who has been an IDDM patient for nearly 40 years. He has become increasingly forgetful and indeed she confides that he took early retirement because blunting of intellect had made it increasingly difficult for him to cope at work. He has always had good diabetic control and rarely reported hypoglycaemic episodes to his doctors. His wife reports however that he took pride in running his sugars low and almost daily required to take additional snacks to ward off hypoglycaemia. In more recent years he had lost the warning signs of hypoglycaemia and had suffered many severe hypoglycaemic episodes requiring aid from his family to bring him round. He feared the loss of his driving licence and had failed to report these incidents to his GP. His wife wonders whether the repeated episodes of hypoglycaemia might have been responsible for his intellectual deterioration.

The fear of hypoglycaemia in the IDDM patient can often be intense and of much greater relevance than the fear of diabetic complications developing at some distant time in the future. Patients may prefer to 'run their sugars a bit high' rather than risk the embarrassment or social consequences of having a 'hypo' at school, work or while driving. Many patients fear the risk of dying during a hypoglycaemic episode or of developing brain damage as a consequence of re-current hypoglycaemias.

Mechanisms underlying hypoglycaemia

Abnormal lowering of blood glucose causes firstly stimulation of the sympathetic nervous system and then progressive depression of brain function.

Autonomic stimulation

Hypoglycaemia stimulates the sympathetic nervous system and also causes release of adrenaline from the adrenal glands. This in turn results in the clinical signs and symptoms of hypoglycaemia including pallor, sweating and tachycardia. A list of adrenergic symptoms caused by hypoglycaemia is given in Box 8.3.

Neuroglycopenia

Glucose is essential to maintain the normal metabolism within brain cells. Severe and prolonged hypoglycaemia will result in a gradual deterioration in brain function. Patients may experience symptoms of numbness or paraesthesia, dizziness and lightheadedness, altered behaviour and deterioration in conscious level until coma develops (Box 8.3).

Treatment of hypoglycaemia

The prevention of severe hypoglycaemia requires the recognition of the early signs by the patient or family members and knowledge of

---

Box 8.3 Symptoms of hypoglycaemia. Those symptoms which cannot easily be allocated to one single group are shown in both columns. Brackets indicate a weak association

Autonomic	Neuroglycopenic
Sweating	Dizziness/feeling faint
Trembling	Confusion
Palpitations	
Warmness	Tiredness
Anxiety	Difficulty with speaking
Nausea	Headache
Tingling of lips, tongue or fingers	Inability to concentrate
Hunger	(Hunger)
(Blurred vision)	Blurred vision
Drowsiness	Drowsiness
Weakness	Weakness
Pallor	Coma
Death is possible	Irritability
	Aggression
	Death is possible

the correct treatment to abort the attack. Patient education is therefore a vital first step in the management of hypoglycaemia, and the primary health care team should be involved in such education. The treatment of hypoglycaemia is discussed more fully in Chapter 10.

Hypoglycaemia: brain damage and death

There is no doubt that severe hypoglycaemia in the neonate causes damage to the developing brain resulting in reduction in IQ and cognitive function. Similarly hypoglycaemia occurring in children who have developed diabetes before the age of 5 or 6 years is likely to impair the intelligence of the child. For this reason tight metabolic control should not be the aim in such young children (Ch. 5).

The effects of severe or repeated hypoglycaemia upon the adult brain are much less certain. Some studies have suggested that mild impairment of IQ or memory can occur, while other studies have been unable to show significant effects of hypoglycaemia. The adult diabetic may have other reasons for deterioration in brain function; micro- and macrovascular disease of the brain or neuropathy involving brain neurones. It is therefore difficult to determine the effects of hypoglycaemia in isolation from these other disease processes.

Insulin overdose is however known to cause both death and severe and permanent brain damage. There is therefore no doubt that in the extreme case, hypoglycaemia can be serious and life-threatening. Similarly, hypoglycaemia in the elderly patient on sulphonylurea therapy can be prolonged and associated with significant risk of mortality (Ch. 4).

The possibility of death during hypoglycaemia worries many patients and their relatives. Most health care professionals would seek to reassure their patients that such deaths are very rare and only occur in patients who take poor care of their diabetes, are alcoholic or have taken deliberate overdoses of insulin. The exact incidence of death due to hypoglycaemia is however not known. Guidance for patients on hypoglycaemia should therefore be balanced and not alarmist.

The anxious wife of the bank manager should be encouraged to bring her husband to the surgery. It is important that other causes of intellectual impairment are excluded, in particular hypothyroidism, vitamin B_{12} deficiency or other metabolic disorders. It should be explained to the patient and his wife that there is no clear evidence that recurrent hypoglycaemia affects mental function. However it would be sensible to relax his metabolic control in the face of hypo-glycaemia unawareness. Clinical examination to identify neurological signs of multiple cerebral infarcts would be important and a CT brain scan may confirm the presence of general cerebral atrophy.

THE ANNUAL REVIEW

From all that has been discussed above it is clear that the com-plications of diabetes pose ominous problems not only for the diabetic patient but also for the health care professionals who look after such patients. There are obvious benefits in screening to prevent complica-tions or to treat the early manifestations and prevent progression of complications. Responsibility for screening lies either with the Primary Health Care Team or the Hospital Team.

Some Primary Health Care Teams will be happy to carry out the full review while others may prefer that the local Hospital Diabetic Team takes responsibility for this. Either way it is important that the GP and the diabetic consultant communicate regarding this vital part of care.

The concept has gradually developed of the 'Annual Review' (the 'MOT'): a single visit per year when screening for complications is undertaken. This visit may or may not be separate from the routine clinic visit. A protocol should be established for the review visit which can guarantee that all necessary procedures are completed. Both in general practice and in hospital diabetic clinics, computerised patient registers are allowing recording of these screening proce-dures and subsequent audit to take place (Ch. 11).

The problem of the social and personal burden of diabetic com-plications was addressed by interested professionals who met in St Vincent, Italy in 1989. From this meeting arose the St Vincent Declaration. This document recommends the establishment of mechanisms for reducing the incidence of diabetic complications. It also sets specific targets for these reductions (Box 8.4). The St Vincent Declaration is discussed more fully in Chapter 12.

The protocol for performing an annual review is provided in Box 8.5. If hypertension or hyperlipidaemia is identified repeat testing is required, and if confirmed, suitable treatment should be started. Further referrals to chiropodist, vascular surgeon or ophthalmologist may be indicated.

Box 8.4   Targets of the St Vincent Declaration

- Reduce new blindness due to diabetes by one third or more.
- Reduce numbers of people entering end-stage diabetic renal failure by at least one third.
- Reduce by one half the rate of limb amputations for diabetic gangrene.
- Cut the morbidity and mortality from coronary heart disease in the diabetic by vigorous programmes of risk factor reduction.
- Achieve pregnancy outcome in the diabetic woman that approximates that of the nondiabetic woman.

A more detailed summary of the St Vincent Declaration is given in Box 12.2, page 258.

Box 8.5   Suggested protocol for the Annual Review

1. Weigh patient and record BMI.
2. Measure blood pressure.
3. Test urine for glucose and protein (albustix).
4. Check visual acuity and undertake fundoscopy through dilated pupils (using 1% tropicamide eye drops).
5. Examine feet: general condition of skin and nails
                   bone deformities
                   peripheral pulses
                   light touch, pin-prick sensation (possibly other
                       sensory tests).
6. Record the following: smoking habits
                           drinking habits
                           attendance at chiropodist.
7. Discuss diabetic control problems: hypoglycaemia/hyperglycaemia and assess self-monitoring skills and recording of results.
8. Audit patient injection techniques and inspect injection sites.
9. Blood for glucose, glycated haemoglobin, urea and electrolytes, lipid profile.
10. Urine for microalbuminuria (patients under 65 years).

SUMMARY

If the targets set by the St Vincent Declaration are to be met, systems for regular screening for diabetic complications must be established. This can either be carried out in the Primary Health Care setting or at the Hospital Diabetic Clinic. Screening will usually be performed at a single annual review visit supported by a computerised patient record system so that recall, follow-up and audit can be implemented. Education of the patient is vital and the importance of alteration in lifestyle to reduce the risk of long-term complications must be emphasised.

REFERENCES

Andersen A R, Christiansen J S, Andersen J K, Kreiner S, Deckert T 1983 Diabetic nephropathy in Type 1 (insulin-dependent) diabetes: an epidemiological study. Diabetologia 25:496–501

Ballard D J, Humphrey L L, Melton L J et al 1988 Epidemiology of persistent proteinuria in type II diabetes mellitus: population-based study in Rochester, Minnesota. Diabetes 37:405–412

Bjorck S, Mulec H, Johnsen S A, Norden G, Aurell M 1992 Renal protective effect of enalapril in diabetic nephropathy. British Medical Journal 304:340–343

Chokroverty S 1982 Proximal nerve dysfunction in diabetic proximal amyotrophy: electrophysiology and electron microscopy. Archives of Neurology 39:403

Davies E G, Petty R G, Kohner E M 1989 Long term effectiveness of photocoagulation for diabetic retinopathy. Eye 3:764–767

The DCCT Research Group 1993 The effect of intensive treatment of diabetes on the development and progression of long-term complications in insulin-dependent diabetes mellitus. New England Journal of Medicine 329:977–986

Donahue R P, Orchard T V 1992 Diabetes mellitus and macrovascular complications. An epidemiological perspective. Diabetes Care 15:1141–1155

Fairburn C G, McCulloch D K, Wu F C 1982 The effects of diabetes on male sexual function. Journal of Clinical Endocrinology and Metabolism 11:749–767

Fields H L (ed) 1990 Pain syndromes in neurology. Butterworth, London

Foulds W S, MacCuish A, Barrie T et al 1983 Diabetic retinopathy in the West of Scotland: its detection and prevalence, and the cost-effectiveness of a proposed screening. Health Bulletin (Edinburgh) 41:318–326

Frick M H, Elo O, Heinonen O P et al 1987 Helsinki Heart Study: primary-prevention trial with gemfibrozil in middle aged men with dyslipidemia. New England Journal of Medicine 317:1237–1245

Hepburn D A, Deary I J, Frier B M, Patrick A W, Quinn J D, Fisher B M 1991 Symptoms of acute insulin-induced hypoglycaemia in humans with and without IDDM: factor analysis approach. Diabetes Care 14:949–957

Hjermann I 1981 The effect of diet and smoking intervention on the incidence of coronary heart disease: report of the Oslo Study Group of a randomised trial in healthy men. Lancet II:1303–1310

Kaplan N M 1989 The deadly quartet. Upper-body obesity, glucose intolerance, hypertriglyceridemia and hypertension. Archives of Internal Medicine 149:1514–1520

Klein B E K, Moss S E, Klein R 1987 Longitudinal measure of glycaemic control and diabetic retinopathy. Diabetes Care 10: 272–277

Krolewski A S, Warram J H, Christlieb A R, Busick E J, Kahn C R 1985 The changing natural history of nephropathy in type 1 diabetes. American Journal of Medicine 78: 785–794

Krans H M J, Porta M, Keen H, Staehr Johansen K 1995 Diabetes care and research in Europe: the St Vincent Declaration action programme. Implementation document. World Health Organization, Rome

Kvinesdal B, Molin J, Froland A, Gram L F 1984 Imipramine treatment of painful diabetic neuropathy. Journal of the American Medical Association 251: 1727–1730

Mogensen C E 1982 Longterm antihypertensive treatment inhibiting progression of diabetic nephropathy. British Medical Journal 304:340–343

Mogensen C E, Schmitz O 1988 Diabetic kidney: from hyperfiltration and microalbuminuria to end-stage renal failure. Medical Clinics of North America 72:1465–1492

Orchard T J, Strandness D E 1993 Assessment of peripheral vascular disease in diabetes. Report and recommendations of an international workshop. Diabetes Care 16:1199–1209

Parving H H, Oxenboll B, Svendsen P Aa, Sandahl Christiansen J, Andersen A R 1982 Early detection of patients at risk of developing diabetic neuropathy. A longitudinal study of urinary albumin excretion. Acta Endocrinologica 100:550–555

Parving H H, Andersen A R, Smidt U M, Hommel E, Mathiesen E R, Svendsen P A 1987 Effect of antihypertensive treatment on kidney function in diabetic nephropathy. British Medical Journal 294:1443–1447

Reaven G M 1988 Role of insulin resistance in human disease. Diabetes 37:1595–1607

Sullivan P M, Caldwell G, Alexandra N, Kohner E M 1990 Long term outcome after photocoagulation for preproliferative diabetic retinopathy. Diabetic Medicine 7:788–794

Viberti G G, Hill R D, Jarret R J, Argyropoulos A, Mahmud U, Keen H 1982 Microalbuminuria as a predictor of clinical nephropathy in insulin-dependent diabetes mellitus. Lancet 1430–1432

Viberti G G, Mogensen C E, Groop L C, Pauls J F 1994 Effect of captopril on progression to chemical proteinuria in patients with insulin-dependent diabetes mellitus and microalbuminuria. Journal of the American Medical Association 271:275–279

West K M 1971 Epidemiology of diabetes and vascular lesions. Elsevier, New York

Williams I, Mayer R F 1976 Subacute proximal diabetic neuropathy. Neurology 26:108

Young M J, Boulton A J M, MacLeod A F, Williams D R R, Sonksen P H 1993 A multicentre study of the prevalence of diabetic peripheral neuropathy in the United Kingdom hospital clinic population. Diabetologia 36:150–154

Zeller K, Whittaker E, Sullivan L, Raskin P, Jacobson H R 1991 Effect of restricting dietary protein on the progression of renal failure in patients with insulin-dependent diabetes mellitus. New England Journal of Medicine 324:78–84

Foot health education

Christine Skinner

■ CONTENTS

INTRODUCTION

The foot is a complex structure which is not only responsible for loco-motion but is also designed to withstand the stresses of body weight whilst walking and standing. These stresses can be responsible for microtrauma that may lead to foot lesions. Foot problems are still the most common cause of hospital admissions for diabetic patients in the United Kingdom and the length of stay is greater than for any other diabetic complication (Williams 1985).

In 1989 there were 696 major amputations performed on diabetic patients in England alone (Dept of Health 1989) and in Scotland in 1993, 36 amputations were carried out as a result of diabetic gangrene affecting the foot. This accounted for a total of 1443 occupied bed days (Common Services Agency 1993).

Most community nurses will be familiar with caring for the diabetic foot. There are two aspects of foot care: assessing the foot and treating foot lesions. Both these aspects are pertinent to the diabetic and to community nurses, and will be considered separately.

The management of the patient should always have a multidisciplinary approach with close liaison between chiropodist, diabetologist, general practitioner, diabetic nurse specialist, the community nurse and footwear specialist.

Treatment by a chiropodist is free to all diabetic patients within the United Kingdom. The chiropodist should be involved in the care of the diabetic soon after diagnosis and thereafter as the patient is referred to them. It is recommended that diabetic patients only attend a State Registered Chiropodist.

FOOT HEALTH EDUCATION

Foot health education plays an important part in any successful management strategy. Patients who have had diabetes for many years may be unaware of the potential problems which can affect their feet. It must be remembered that whilst the patient should be aware of these problems it is important that the patient is not caused unnecessary alarm. It is essential therefore to gain the patient's confidence and trust and establish a rapport. In so doing the practitioner is able to gauge the levels of knowledge and understanding the patient may have. Reassurance is essential to minimise the patient's anxiety and re-enforcement of foot health education encourages good patient compliance.

ASSESSMENT OF THE DIABETIC FOOT

Community nurses will be involved in assessing the foot for diabetic complications as part of the annual screening visit and as part of their everyday care for their patients. General practitioners may also assess the feet at the screening clinic.

Prior to examining the feet, certain facts should be ascertained:

- duration of diabetes
- does the patient have NIDDM or IDDM?
- present level of control
- do they experience pain or cramping in their legs when walking?
- do they have a numbness or tingling sensation in their feet?

- has there been any history of foot ulceration?
- does the patient smoke?

Foot assessment requires some skills and experience in examining and interpretation. Community nurses should therefore be supervised by their GPs until the GP has deemed them competent. Examination of the foot involves assessment of soft tissues, structural deformities, vascular and neurological status.

Soft tissue assessment

This involves assessing both the skin and the nails.

Skin

When assessing the colour of the skin a comparison of the feet should be made. The colour and temperature of the skin are indicative of the blood flow through the foot. The skin of a foot with a good blood flow will be pale pink and warm to touch. If there is impaired blood flow the skin will be cold and pale. Cyanosis indicates a poor oxygen content and therefore poor blood supply. The appearance of a cold, hyperaemic (bright red) foot demonstrates ischaemia to the peripheral tissues and should be considered as a potential problem. The skin of an ischaemic foot is shiny, stretched, hairless and cool to touch.

The foot should be examined for the presence of soft tissue lesions such as callus, corns and any abrasions or indications of trauma. The interdigital spaces are often macerated and are a potential site for fungal infection.

Patients with autonomic neuropathy will have decreased sweating which results in dry, devitalised skin. The plantar aspect of the foot and the heel area are often affected, with the posterior aspect of the heel liable to fissuring.

Nails

The nails may vary in appearance depending on the vascular state of the foot. In the ischaemic foot the nails may be thickened and slow growing. If they are infected by fungi they will appear thickened, discoloured and have a 'musty' smell (Fig. 9.1). The nail grooves should also be examined to ensure there is no callus or small spike of nail which has penetrated the soft tissues of the groove, which can lead to an infected ingrowing toenail (Fig. 9.2).

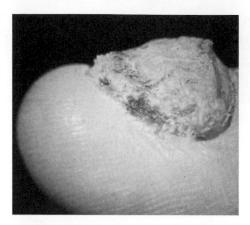

Fig. 9.1 The diabetic foot: nails thickened and discoloured by fungal infection.

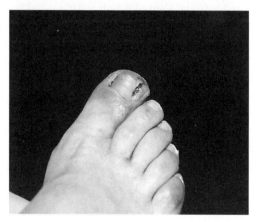

Fig. 9.2 Infected ingrowing toenail.

Structural deformities

Structural deformities as a complication of diabetes act as a potential site for ulceration because the area is subjected to abnormal stresses.

The toes are often in a clawed position as a result of motor neuropathy which causes wasting of the small intrinsic muscles and allows the long flexors to have an unopposed action (Fig. 9.3). The metatarsal heads therefore become much more prominent on the plantar surface and are subjected to greater stress during walking.

Structural deformities may also be present in the diabetic foot as a

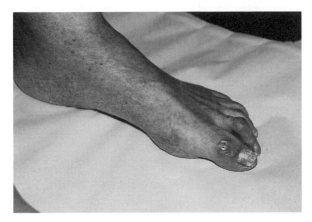

Fig. 9.3 Clawing of the toes as a result of motor neuropathy: long flexor muscles have unopposed action because small intrinsic muscles are wasted.

result of changes from Charcot neuropathic joints. These changes are frequently associated with full sensory neuropathy and often follow trauma to the foot (Boehm 1962).

Vascular assessment

The diabetic foot can be affected by both macrovascular and microvascular disease. Both have significant influences on the clinical appearance and the subsequent management of the foot. Symptoms of vascular insufficiency should be elicited from the patient. If the patient complains of intermittent claudication, its severity can be assessed by determining how far the patient can walk before symptoms develop. It is also necessary to determine if the patient suffers from rest pain, an indication of severe ischaemia.

It is essential to distinguish the pain of ischaemia from that of neuropathy, which may present as a burning sensation.

Clinical assessment of the vascular state may be carried out routinely by performing a variety of physical tests. All members of the health care team, after suitable training, could perform these tests.

Physical tests

Palpation of pulses

Peripheral circulation can be assessed by palpation of pedal pulses (Fig. 9.4).

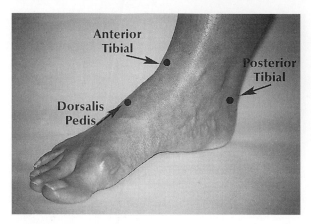

Fig. 9.4   Palpation of pedal pulses.

Dorsalis Pedis artery is a continuation of the Anterior Tibial artery and the pulse can be palpated on the dorsal aspect of the foot in the region of the intermediate cuneiform.

Anterior Tibial pulse can be palpated on the front of the ankle midway between the two malleoli.

Posterior Tibial pulse can be palpated immediately behind the medial malleolus.

Whilst confidence is essential in palpating pedal pulses, such confidence is only acquired through practice. All members of the health care team are encouraged to develop this skill with normal, healthy people before progressing to patients with known vascular complications.

It should be noted however that arteriovenous shunts will develop due to autonomic neuropathy and as a result, blood flow bypasses the capillary bed. Thus patients may have bounding arterial pulses but have poor blood supply to the surrounding tissues. This is responsible for the venous engorgement often seen on the dorsum of the foot (Ward & Boulton 1987).

Temperature gradient

The temperature gradient can be assessed by gently running the back of the hand from below the knee distally to the toes. If there are any obvious changes intra and inter limb, these should be noted.

Capillary refill

This is assessed by gently pressing the plantar aspect of the hallux until it blanches. Pressure is removed and the tissues allowed to reperfuse. Normal capillary refill should be 3 seconds.

Presence or absence of oedema
The presence of oedema can prevent the palpation of pedal pulses. If present, the affected sites should be noted.

Presence or absence of varicose veins
Varicose veins can lead to oedema of the ankle or dorsum of the foot and create a problem with socks and shoes.

Neurological assessment
Neuropathy is a major contributory factor in the development of ulceration in the diabetic foot (Thomson et al 1991). The patient suffering from neuropathy may present with two contrasting symptoms. They may complain of pain and paraesthesia, or of numbness with loss of pain and loss of temperature appreciation. If the patient complains of pain it is important to distinguish the pain from that of ischaemia by assessing the quality of the pain and by examining the peripheral circulation. The paraesthesia may be a tingling or burning sensation or the patient may describe a hypersensitivity on contact.

If there is neuropathy present then a thorough structural assessment must be performed. This determines areas of pressure which may result in the development of callus and corns and eventually ulcers.

Neuropathy may also result in damage to the soft tissue of the foot because having lost sensation, the patient is unaware of trauma to the foot. Hence patients are advised not to walk around on bare feet (Boxes 9.1 and 9.2).

Light touch
This can be assessed using a piece of cotton wool. The patient's foot is gently touched with the cotton wool and sites identified where it can/cannot be appreciated. This commences distally and moves proximally, thereby moving from a potentially numb area to a sensory area. It is easier to identify the boundary of sensory loss when moving from a numb area to an area of normal sensation. The patient should have his/her eyes closed during this examination. Ensure that there is minimal variation in the pressure of application of the cotton wool.

Sharp and blunt sensation
A Neurotip can be used to identify if this sensation is present or absent.

Box 9.1   Foot health education for the healthy diabetic

- Never walk barefoot.
- Change hosiery daily.
- Inspect feet daily for corns/callosities/plantar warts/athlete's foot.
- If any of the above are present they should only be treated by a State Registered Chiropodist.
- With the slightest abrasion or infection in your feet, contact your GP, community nurse, diabetic nurse specialist, diabetic consultant or chiropodist.
- Never use proprietary treatments for callus or corns, as they contain acids.
- Cut toe nails straight across.
- Purchase new shoes from a shop which will measure your feet and fit the shoes for you.
- Never wear new shoes for a long period of time.
- Stop smoking.
- Only attend a State Registered Chiropodist.

Box 9.2   Foot health education for the 'at risk' diabetic foot

Box 9.1 plus the undernoted:
- Wash feet daily.
- Do not cut your own toe nails.
- Inspect feet daily for any open lesions, cracking, dryness, change in colour, swelling, corn, callus, blisters, warts or signs of infection.
- Use a mirror to inspect the soles of your feet or ask someone to look for you.
- Only use a hot water bottle to heat your bed–never place it next to your feet.
- Never sit close to the fire or heater.
- Check inside shoes for foreign objects.
- Wear shoes with soft uppers, preferably lacing.
- Never wear garters to hold up stockings or socks.
- Attend a State Registered Chiropodist regularly.

Again the patient's eyes should be closed during this examination and the assessor should commence distally and work proximally.

Autonomic neuropathy

The skin will appear dry and flaky with perhaps fissuring in the heel area. This can be a potential site for bacterial infection.

There are other tests requiring specialised equipment which can be used to enhance the examination of the diabetic foot. These are usually carried out by the chiropodist.

The purpose of assessing the diabetic foot under the various parameters outlined above is to determine the foot which is 'at risk' of developing callus, corns and ulcers.

The 'at risk' foot may therefore be defined as the foot which has any one of the clinical signs detailed in Box 9.3.

Further detailed instructions in foot health care (Box 9.2) should be given if the patient is assessed as having an 'at risk' foot. Patient education in the prevention of foot problems is the first line of defence. The patient's ability to understand the importance of foot health education should be assessed. The patient should also receive regular chiropody care and be made aware of a system for seeking immediate medical attention if a foot problem arises. All health care professionals must continually reinforce appropriate foot health education.

TREATMENT AND MANAGEMENT OF FOOT LESIONS

Patients may present with a wide range of foot problems. Some patients only require routine nail cutting and simple advice on foot care (Box 9.1). Others will have nail problems, callus, corns or even ulceration and will require more intensive care and education (Box 9.2).

Nail reduction

While nurses are not advised to cut the toe nails of the diabetic patient, they may teach the able diabetic safe practice in nail care. This only applies to patients with healthy feet. Those 'at risk' must attend a chiropodist regularly for nail routine.

Box 9.3 The 'at risk' foot has any one of these clinical signs

- ischaemia
- numbness
- structural deformities
- callus and/or corn
- absence of pedal pulses
- a capillary refill time in excess of 3 seconds
- limb pain and/or paraesthesia
- intermittent claudication
- history of foot ulcers
- loss of sensation of light touch, sharp and blunt touch

Nails should be cut straight across without cutting down into the corners. Check that there are no ragged edges or sharp corners which could irritate either the soft tissues of the sulcus of the nail or the adjacent toe. Small spurs of nail may penetrate the soft tissues of the sulcus and an ingrowing toe nail may develop (Fig. 9.2).

If the nail is excessively curved a light pack of sterile cotton wool or chamois can be used under the lateral edge of the nail to prevent it irritating the soft tissues of the sulcus (Fig. 9.5).

If the nails are thickened as a result of trauma or peripheral vascular disease the patient should be referred to a chiropodist.

Callus and corns

Diabetic patients are advised never to treat callus or corns with proprietary medication. 'Corn pads' contain salicylic acid which may cause chemical trauma to the foot. This is undesirable especially if the patient has neuropathy. These lesions should only be treated by a State Registered Chiropodist.

Padding and strapping

The chiropodist will reduce the callus and corn, to minimise the pressure being exerted onto the area, and provide padding and strapping.

Footwear

Ill-fitting footwear can contribute to foot problems such as ulceration in the diabetic patient (Thomson et al 1991). Footwear should be adequate to

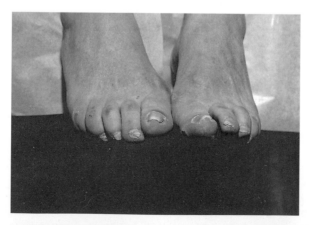

Fig. 9.5   Nail reduction: sterile cotton wool used under lateral edge of the nail to prevent irritation.

accommodate the shape of the foot. Patients with healthy feet and no lesions can be advised to purchase shoes from a reputable retailer where their feet will be measured and shoes fitted prior to purchase.

Footwear should also be appropriate to the lifestyle of the patient. Good quality training shoes are ideal for the patient who is involved in walking a great deal as this type of footwear has a deep toe box and thick cushioned sole.

Female patients should be advised on the limited use of court shoes which are constricting to the toes and have no retaining strap. The height of the heel results in the weight being concentrated onto the forefoot.

Patients with foot deformities such as hallux valgus, hammer or claw toes require shoes which are wider and deeper than normal. These can be provided from a number of specialist footwear suppliers and are available on the NHS (Fig. 9.6). Patients with gross foot deformities will require custom-made shoes which can be authorised by the patient's GP, orthopaedic surgeon or diabetic consultant. Some patients will require insoles to alleviate abnormal pressures in the foot. Again, the chiropodist can facilitate and supervise these.

INFECTION

Poorly controlled diabetic patients are more susceptible to infections, and if ulceration is present are likely to have delayed healing.

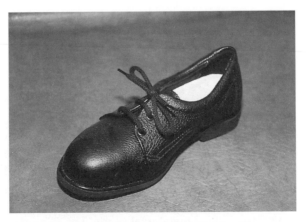

Fig. 9.6   Footwear for patients with foot deformities.

Fungal infection

The most common site on the foot for fungal infection is the interdigital spaces. The skin in the affected area may be white, macerated and peeling. The patient will complain of itching and there is the danger of the patient scratching the area and spreading the infection on to the dorsum of the foot. Treatment is usually easy when the fungus responsible has been identified and antifungal agents commenced. However, as with nondiabetic patients, fungal infections tend to recur.

When dealing with this type of infection it is important to stress to the patient the need for good foot hygiene and that they avoid scratching as this may break the skin allowing a secondary bacterial infection to develop. The patient should be referred to their GP for antibiotic therapy should this occur.

Bacterial infection

Secondary infection can be a common problem following tissue break-down in the diabetic foot. The most common organisms responsible are staphylococci, beta-haemolytic streptococci, aerobic Gram-negative bacilli and anaerobic bacteria (Edmonds et al 1986). When the patient presents with a discharging lesion a swab of the pus should be taken and sent to bacteriology. The patient should be referred immediately to their GP for antibiotic cover. Localised treatment involves cleansing the wound with sterile, normal saline and dressing with an appropriate dressing (Fig. 9.7) as well as providing protection to the area. The area is monitored for signs of cellulitis and lymphangitis. X-ray of the foot is important to exclude gas gangrene or osteomyelitis.

Close liaison with all those involved in the treatment of the patient enables a satisfactory outcome.

ULCERATION

Abnormal foot pressures are a contributory factor in the development of ulceration in the diabetic foot (Masson et al 1989). Clinical evaluation identifies areas of abnormally high pressure which may result in the development of corn and callus. There is an increased risk of ulceration developing if callus is not reduced, if pressure persists, or if the foot has diminished sensation.

The most common sites are the dorsum of the toes if they are clawed, and the plantar aspect of the metatarsal heads. This clinical evaluation is

Is the ulcer

Black & necrotic	Yes →	1 Refer to GP/Diabetologist 2 Apply dry sterile dressing

No ↓

Yellow & sloughy	Yes →	1 Debride surrounding callous 2 Irrigate with normal, sterile saline 3 Intrasite Gel Granuflex

No ↓

Exuding	Yes →	1 Irrigate with normal sterile saline 2 Light/med: Intrasite Gel Granuflex 3 Heavy: Iodosorb

No ↓

Infection	Yes →	1 Refer for antibiotic cover 2 Irrigate with normal, sterile saline 3 Inadine or suitable antiseptic

No ↓

Malodorous	Yes →	1 Irrigate with normal, sterile saline 2 Lyofoam

No ↓

Granulating	Yes →	1 Irrigate with normal, sterile saline 2 Granuflex

No ↓

Epithelialising	Yes →	1 Irrigate with normal, sterile saline 2 Inadine Granuflex

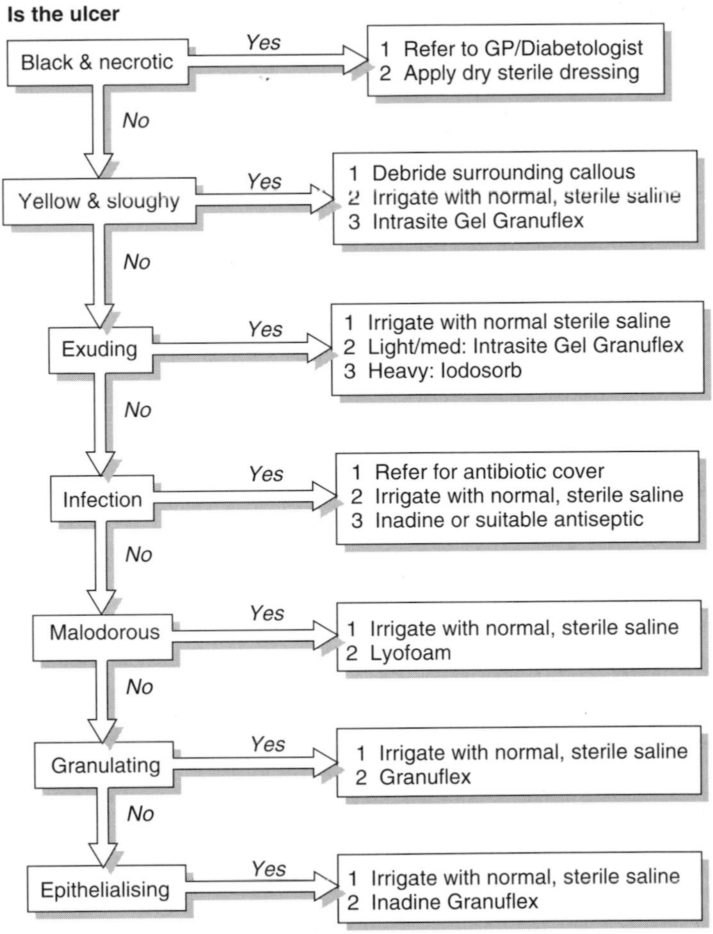

Fig. 9.7 Diabetic foot ulcer protocol.

particularly important if there is neuropathy or vascular disease present (Box 9.3).

Ulceration can also develop in the diabetic foot as a result of constant pressure, e.g. poorly fitting shoes or a foreign object in the shoe. A patient affected by peripheral neuropathy causing loss of sensation will allow the pressure to continue for many hours, unaware of tissue damage.

The clinical appearance of the ulcerated area must be recorded to allow objective assessment of healing, by serial measurement of ulcer size. This can be achieved by using a ruler, trace if necessary, or if possible a photograph of the area and surrounding tissue.

The patient should be referred to his/her diabetic consultant for initiation of treatment if an ulcer is present. Community nurses will then be advised regarding wound protocols.

Relieving pressure on an ulcer

To assist in the healing process, the wound must not be subjected to any unnecessary trauma or excessive, abnormal weight-bearing stresses. Complete bed rest is often desirable but not always practical or acceptable to the patient. Therefore alternative regimes should be considered. Chiropodial techniques can play an important role in this aspect of management of diabetic ulceration.

Suitable footwear should be sufficiently wide and deep to accommodate any foot deformity. It should also have a retaining medium such as laces or 'T' bar. Patients should be advised on the need for such footwear.

An alternative option for the patient is a walking plaster cast which relieves pressure on the affected area but allows them to remain mobile (Pollard & Le Quesne 1983). This is called a 'Scotchcast Boot' which is often adopted and consists of a lightly padded boot enclosed in a fibreglass tape shell (Fig. 9.8). Some patients have found these casts cumber-

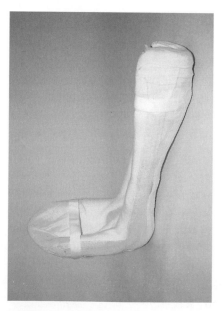

Fig. 9.8 The 'Scotchcast Boot'.

some. They are contraindicated if severe infection is present or if there is peripheral ischaemia.

The 'Hope Removal Walking Cast' has been devised by a team working with diabetic patients (Williams 1994). It meets the objectives of keeping weight from the plantar ulceration and has the advantage over the 'Scotchcast Boot' in that it is removable allowing dressings to be changed. It is also cosmetically more acceptable to the patient (Fig. 9.9).

Alternatively a moulded insole can be manufactured to prevent excessive weightbearing on the ulcerated site (Fig. 9.10).

CLINICAL APPEARANCE OF ULCERS

Neuropathic ulcers

A remarkably accurate description of a neuropathic ulcer was first given

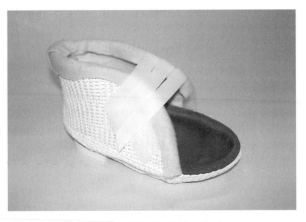

Fig. 9.9 The Hope Removable Walking Cast.

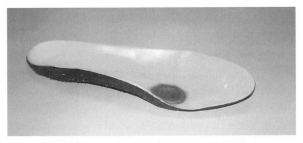

Fig. 9.10 A moulded insole to prevent excessive pressure on a foot ulcer.

as long ago as 1818, 'a round ulcer in the sole of the foot surrounded by a remarkably rough hardening of thick cuticle . . . characterised by a great degree of insensitivity' (Mott 1818).

Neuropathic ulcers characteristically develop on areas of abnormal pressure such as the plantar aspect of the metatarsal heads. Ulceration can also develop on the medial side of the first metatarsal or lateral side of the fifth metatarsal as a result of pressure from shoes.

The ulcer often has a 'punched out' appearance and consists of a central cavity, usually much larger than the opening into it, surrounded by a hard thick plaque of hyperkeratotic tissue. The ulcer may have slough present on the base or have an infected pus discharge with or without surrounding cellulitis.

Characteristically it is painless, and often a moist discharge on hosiery alerts the patient to the lesion. The foot is often warm, pink and dry with palpable pedal pulses.

The neuropathic foot is also at risk of ulceration from direct trauma, e.g. standing on sharp objects; thermal trauma, e.g. hot water bottles; chemical trauma, e.g. 'corn pads' which contain salicylic acid. This is why the diabetic patient is advised never to use these products.

Case Study 9.1

A 64-year-old housewife who has had NIDDM for 10 years has been meticulous about her diet and control since diagnosis. She attends the diabetic clinic for annual review and regularly attends the chiropodist to have her nails cut, having no other foot pathologies. On a routine visit to the clinic she complains of numbness in her right foot.

On closer inspection of the foot there is a small ulcer under the second metatarsal head and evidence of leakage on her tights. The woman is adamant that she never walks barefooted and only ever wears the lacing shoe she had with her. The shoe is examined to reveal a drawing pin sticking through the sole of her right shoe. It was unclear how long it had been there as the patient had not checked the inside of her shoe for several days.

From the development of this lesion and the history it was obvious that this woman had developed peripheral neuropathy.

Tests were carried out by the diabetic consultant to determine its extent. As on all visits the patient's circulation was assessed by checking pedal pulses, colour, capillary refill and temperature gradient. These latter tests were satisfactory. She was immediately referred to the chiropodist.

The chiropodist, aware that the patient had now developed peripheral neuropathy, proceeded to dress the ulcer. The foot was cleansed with antiseptic solution and the ulcer was debrided using a scalpel. All dressings should be considered as sterile dressings whether done in a clinic setting or in the patient's home. An assessment of the ulcer was made regarding size and condition of the base. As there was a discharge and surrounding inflammation a swab was taken of the exudate and sent for culture and sensitivity. As the wound was showing signs of infection and there was slough at the base, an appropriate dressing was selected (Fig. 9.7). The ulcer was irrigated with sterile, normal saline and gently dried using sterile gauze. The area was dressed and a deflective felt pad applied.

The drawing pin was removed from her shoe and the patient's GP contacted to inform him of the situation and to request antibiotic therapy. A further appointment was made for the next day and the patient advised to elevate the foot and reduce weight-bearing as far as possible.

As this woman had now developed peripheral neuropathy she required further foot health education which could be provided by the chiropodist.

On the subsequent visit the dressing was removed and the area assessed. There was evidence of discharge. The area was irrigated with sterile, normal saline. The base of the ulcer was cleaner but there was still evidence of slough. A further dressing was applied and the patient asked to return the next day. The patient was then closely monitored until the ulcer healed. Her diabetic consultant was kept informed of the developments in her condition.

The long-term management of this patient would be to re-educate her in foot health education and continue to see her at the clinic at regular intervals.

Ischaemic ulcers

Ischaemic ulcers may develop on the foot of the diabetic patient suffering from peripheral vascular disease. They can develop on the dorsum or apices of the toes, or the outer borders of the foot. This is particularly so if hallux valgus is present, the forefoot is broad and the patient wears tight-fitting shoes.

Ischaemic necrosis of the tissue may develop as a result of pressure of the footwear obliterating the capillary flow to the area, or as a result of a blockage in the vessel to the area.

The area is usually dry and has a definite line of demarcation which is characteristic of gangrene. If the blockage has been acute, oedema and infection will occur giving a wet gangrene. The patient will complain of severe pain and there will be a history of intermittent claudication and rest pain.

Case Study 9.2

The patient is a 45-year-old man who has had IDDM for 30 years. He works as a draughtsman, is relatively inactive and smokes 40 cigarettes a day. He regularly attends the chiropodist for the reduction of a corn on his left foot and to have his toe nails cut. He is aware of the importance of these visits as his circulation has deteriorated over the past year. He initially complained of intermittent claudication after walking a distance of 100 yards but recently this distance has decreased.

He presents to the chiropodist complaining of a small discoloured area at the tip of his left second toe. On examination of his feet, they are pale and cold to touch. Pedal pulses are absent and on questioning he complains of rest pain particularly in bed. He shows signs of further deterioration of the arterial supply to his lower limbs.

The second toe of the left foot is dusky purple at the metatarsal phalangeal joint and gets progressively darker towards the tip, where it is black. The area is dry and shows no sign of any exudate. He complains of severe pain which prevents him from sleeping at night.

The area is swabbed with sterile, normal saline and a dry, sterile dressing applied. His GP is informed of the development in the patient's condition, and immediately refers the patient to his diabetic consultant for further advice. Referral to a vascular surgeon for investigation of the main limb arteries is advisable. Any stenosis present may be amenable to arterial bypass graft to revascularise the lower limb.

The long-term management of this patient involves a combination of monitoring and education. The patient is advised to stop smoking. He will continue to be treated on a regular basis for foot care, and appropriate foot health advice would be reinforced. Footwear advice would also be given and, if necessary, prescribed. The patient would also be encouraged to commence some regular exercise such as a short walk on a daily basis.

CURRENT RECOMMENDATIONS FOR WOUND DRESSINGS

There is great variation and debate in the treatment of both ischaemic and neuropathic ulceration with regard to topical dressing and antibiotic therapy. Treatment therefore will depend very much on the local exper- tise.

Assessment of the wound for dressing

The selection process of the dressing is dependent on the assessment of the wound initially. On examination of the wound it is essential to determine which features are present (Box 9.4).

The wound may have more than one of these features. The dressing of choice should address the most prominent or serious factor in the medical opinion.

If infection is present, a swab must be sent for culture, organism and sensitivity and the patient commenced on antibiotic cover. In diabetics, such antibiotic therapy is often of a much longer duration than in the normal population and cover for periods of several weeks is not unusual.

Wound cleansing is essential before applying any dressing, and sterile, normal saline is the one of choice. The use of chlorinated solutions such as Milton or Eusol are no longer recommended for cleansing wounds. They have been found to be toxic to tissues and cells involved in the healing process. They can be irritants to surrounding healthy tissue and have been known to cause bleeding. Hydrogen peroxide is no longer recommended for irrigation of wounds as it can cause irritation to the tissues, stinging and a burning sensation (Leaper 1986).

There are however a number of wound dressings currently available which have been used with a degree of success depending on the stage of ulceration.

Box 9.4 Determine which features are present prior to wound dressing

- necrosis
- infection
- slough
- granulation

- epithelialisation
- depth
- exudate
- malodour

The use of more traditional dressings such as gauze with antiseptics is less favoured, as fibres from the gauze can remain on the surface acting as an irritant and delay healing. If there is discharge from the wound this may cause adherence of the dressing to the wound surface. Removal of the dressing may further traumatise the healing wound, damaging the granulating tissue.

Interactive dressings

These provide the optimum conditions for wound healing by maintaining a moist environment at the wound surface. They also allow gaseous exchange of oxygen, carbon dioxide and water vapour but are impermeable to the passage of bacteria.

There has been a great deal of controversy as to the use of totally occlusive dressings, preventing the passage of oxygen to the wound. Some research has found that there is rapid formation of capillaries and granulation tissue with an anaerobic environment and as a result of the occlusion, prostaglandin synthesis is inhibited and therefore pain is reduced (Morgan 1990a).

When dealing with diabetic ulceration, however, a great deal of consideration must be given before selecting or applying an occlusive dressing. This should not be used if microvascular disease is present or if anaerobic bacteria infect the wound (Morgan 1990b).

Thermal insulation also aids in the healing process, so dressings should provide insulation and the patient should be encouraged to choose suitable footwear.

Environmental dressings

These dressings tend to be more expensive than the traditional dressings. They can be cost-effective however because they may be left in situ for several days if the wound is clean. This reduces the need to redress a foot on a daily basis, thus decreasing the costs of both materials and time for the chiropodist or community nurse.

There are many types of environmental dressings from which to select. The groups are listed in Box 9.5.

It is essential that the appropriate dressing is chosen depending on the characteristics of the wound. Each group will be considered in turn to allow the reader the opportunity to compare and contrast the advantages and disadvantages of each.

Semi-permeable polymeric films

These are cheap, permeable to water vapour and gases but act as a

Box 9.5 Classification of environmental dressings	
• semi-permeable polymeric films	• dextranomers
• hydrocolloids	• alginates
• hydrogels	• polyurethane foams

barrier to external contamination. They can be left in situ for up to 7 days. There is sometimes however a problem with sizing for smaller wounds and as they are non-absorbant they cannot be used if there is heavy exudate present. Care should be exercised with thin, fragile but intact skin. They are recommended for shallow ulcers with little exudate.

Example: Dermafilm, Dermoclude, Ensure-it, Omiderm, Opsite, Polyskin, Tegaderm

Features: sterile; thin; transparent; hypoallergenic; adhesive film

Uses: shallow ulcers with little exudate

Contraindications: heavily exuding wounds as they may trap the exudate

Requirements: top dressing to protect and insulate the wound.

Hydrocolloids

These dressings are adhesive, flexible and occlusive. They consist of two layers, an outer protective waterproof layer which is bonded to an inner layer of hydrocolloid particles and a hydrophobic polymer.

The inner layer of these dressings absorbs the exudate, swells, liquefies and forms a soft moist yellow gel over the wound surface – THIS SHOULD NOT BE CONFUSED WITH SLOUGH. When removed the gel separates causing no trauma to the tissues. However, care should be taken when removing the dressings as they may damage fragile skin. They encourage formation of granulation tissue but may be malodorous. They are easy to use and allow rapid debridement and, as they are waterproof, allow the patient to bathe.

Examples: Biofilm, Granuflex, Intrasite, Varihesive

Uses: wound requiring debridement of necrotic tissue; moderate exudate

Contraindications: anaerobic bacteria are present in the wound.

Hydrogels

This dressing consists of a pale yellow transparent gel containing starch copolymer. It is available in a single foil sachet or a small plastic dispenser.

Dressings must be changed daily if slough is present but can be left for 3 days in clean wounds. The gel is easy to apply and may reduce pain.

However it may be considered wasteful as the remainder of the dispenser or sachet must be discarded. If the gel is difficult to remove, a soak of sterile, normal saline solution should be used.

Examples: Intrasite (previously Scherisorb Gel)

Indications: sloughy wounds (deep or shallow); granulating wounds; sinuses

Contraindications: do not use with iodine or povidone iodine preparations.

Dextranomers

These dressings are hydrophilic and absorb wound exudate, carrying debris and bacteria away from the wound surface. Some are in granule or bead form and are difficult to apply to the foot. These dressings should never be allowed to dry out and must be changed daily. The area should always be cleansed thoroughly with sterile, normal saline solution.

Examples: Debrisan, Iodosorb

Uses: sloughy, infected, exudating wounds.

Alginates

Manufactured from brown seaweed and available as flat pads, packing or ribbon. These dressings are biodegradable, cheap and easy to apply. They absorb the wound exudate and form a gel which moulds to the shape of the cavity. Dressings should be changed daily if heavy exudate is present or every 3 days if low exudate. To facilitate the removal of the dressing, sterile normal saline solution must be used.

Examples: Kaltostat, Kaltocarb, Kaltoclude, Sorbsan

Indications: use on exuding wounds

Contraindications: dry or necrotic wounds.

Polyurethane foams

Polyurethane foams are manufactured as flat sheets with an outer layer preventing leakage of exudate and an inner surface which is hydrophilic. Some may have a carbon layer which controls offensive odours. These dressings should be changed daily depending on the exudate. As the wound heals and discharge lessens they may be left in place for up to 7 days. They have high thermal properties. Dressing size can be a problem for small areas.

Examples: Lyofoam, Coraderm, Silastic foam

Indications: medium to heavy exuding wounds; malodorous wounds

Contraindications: patients sensitive to nylon.

Prior to the selection of a specific dressing, consideration must be given to both the stage of the wound to be dressed and the various properties of different dressings available. Community nurses who may be responsible for undertaking the dressings should not alter the prescribed dressing without consulting the person who prescribed it.

MANAGEMENT OF FOOT ULCERATION

The management of the diabetic patient's foot can be variable depending on the presenting clinical picture. All involved in the care of these patients should be vigilant to address the following risk factors for development of foot ulceration:

- poor eyesight—unable to cut own toe nails or inspect feet daily
- elderly patient —less mobile to deal with normal foot hygiene
- previous foot ulceration—area of high pressure or fragile skin
- smoking—responsible for vascular disease and resultant effect on blood supply to the foot. Danger of patient burning his/her skin with a cigarette or lighter but being unaware that they have done so due to neuropathy
- neuropathy
- peripheral vascular disease
- structural deformity of the foot.

The multidisciplinary team in community and hospital must work together to prevent foot problems and to treat early any detected abnormalities. The ultimate goal is to keep 'these feet . . . made for walking'.

SUMMARY

Caring for the feet of the diabetic patient is a challenge to the patient and all members of the Health Care Team. Education plays a crucial role in the prevention of foot problems and this must be reinforced consistently by all Health Care Team members.

Daily assessment of the feet by the patient is the first point of prevention. At the slightest irregularity, no matter how trivial it may seem, the patient should consult his/her GP, community nurse, diabetic nurse specialist or chiropodist. Good communications between the multidisciplinary team facilitate speedy management of the diabetic foot.

One stated aim of the St Vincent Declaration is '. . . to raise an awareness in the population and among health care professionals of present opportunities and the future needs for prevention of the complications of diabetes and of diabetes itself, and to reduce the number of amputations for diabetic gangrene in Europe by 50%' (Diabetes Care & Research in Europe 1994).

A multidisciplinary approach will facilitate the achievement of this goal.

REFERENCES

Boehm J J 1962 Diabetic charcot joints. New England Journal of Medicine 267:185
Boulton A J M, Scarpello J H B, Ward J D 1982 Venous oxygenation in the diabetic neuropathic foot: evidence of arteriovenous shunting? Diabetologia 22:6–8
Department of Health–Statistics and Management Information Division, 1989 Amputation Statistics for England, Wales and Northern Ireland. Department of Health, London
Common Services Agency 1993 Scottish medical records information. NHS Scotland, Edinburgh
Diabetes Care and Research in Europe: The Saint Vincent Declaration 1990. Diabetic Medicine 7:360
Edmonds M E, Blundell M P, Morris H E, Maelor-Thomas E, Cotton L T, Watkins P J 1986 Improved survival of the diabetic foot: the role of the specialised foot clinic. Quarterly Journal of Medicine 60:763–771
Leaper D 1986 Antiseptics and their effect on healing tissue. Nursing Times 82:22:45–47
Masson E A, Hay E M, Stockley I, Veves A, Betts R P, Boulton A J M 1989 Abnormal foot pressures alone may not cause ulceration. Diabetic Medicine 6:426–428
Morgan D 1990a Development of a wound management policy: part 1. Pharmaceutical Journal (March):295–297
Morgan D 1990b Development of a wound management policy: part 2. Pharmaceutical Journal (March):358–359
Mott V A 1818 A cause of circular callous ulcer in the bottom of the foot. Medical Surgical Register New York:1:129
Pollard J P, Le Quense L P 1983 Method of healing diabetic forefoot ulcers. British Medical Journal 286:436–437
Thomson F J, Veves A, Ashe H et al 1991 A team approach to diabetic foot care—the Manchester experience. The Foot 1:2:75–82
Ward J D, Boulton A J M 1987 Peripheral vascular abnormalities and diabetic neuropathy. In: Dyck P J et al (eds) Diabetic neuropathy. Saunders, Philadelphia
Williams A 1994 The Hope removable walking cast; a method of treatment for diabetic/neuropathic ulceration. Practical Diabetes 11:1:20–23
Williams D R R 1985 Hospital admissions of diabetic patients: information from hospital activity analysis. Diabetic Medicine 2:27–32

Educating the patient

Joan McDowell

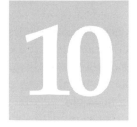

INTRODUCTION

'You can take a horse to the water—but you cannot make him drink.'
A well-known saying which unfortunately describes the whole area
of patient education. However, patient education has always been
fundamental to caring for the patient with diabetes. For many, education was considered to be 'telling' the patient certain facts. The
patient was a passive recipient of information which might or might
not be related to his/her individual lifestyle and hence it had little
application for the patient. This did not allow for patient choice,
participation or the patient's lifestyle.

More recently it has become evident that education should assist
the patient to acquire the right skills to develop appropriate behaviour
and to assert control over factors which affect his/her health. The
role of the nurse is therefore to 'empower' patients with their options
and assist them in making choices which may affect their lifestyle
(Ch. 3).

Patients who predominantly take on the responsibility for their own health are said to have an 'internal' locus of control. Some patients, however, opt not to assume this responsibility for themselves and allow the responsibility for diabetic monitoring and control to fall to the health care team. These patients are referred to as having an 'external' locus of control. A third group of patients believe that control of their diabetes is a matter of pure chance.

In relating this to patient education, those patients who have an internal locus of control will respond to empowerment in education. Those with an external locus of control will be passive recipients of education who may 'follow the basic rules' but will not become actively involved in their self-management. For example, they would probably self-monitor their diabetes but would not necessarily adjust their insulin. The third group of patients are those who appear at a diabetic clinic once every ten years and boast that 'their diabetes causes them no problem'!

Education can be facilitated on a one-to-one basis, in small groups, or in a more formal seminar or discussion group. Teaching may take place in a patient's home, the surgery, a diabetic centre in the community or the hospital. The education may be structured and planned or casual and opportunistic. Materials used for education will include audiovisual material, posters, leaflets, diagrams, practical equipment and where possible, demonstrations.

Unfortunately some of the educational literature available is unsuitable for the elderly or those with impaired visual acuity. Written material used extensively for patient education seldom meets the guidelines for readable print size (Petterson et al 1994). The language used is either too technical or contains jargon which hinders understanding (Overland et al 1993). Health care professionals using literature to support their education sessions must be aware of the problems of readability and literacy status of the material which they use.

These problems are compounded where English is not the patient's first language. There is therefore a considerable need for reading materials which are culturally specific. The British Diabetic Association (BDA) is currently addressing this problem.

At diagnosis, the patient is usually anxious and although appearing keen to learn is not necessarily in the most receptive frame of mind to acquire new knowledge. An education programme must therefore be planned and staged in order to take into account the patient's ability to assimilate information.

The first stage of education commences at the time of diagnosis. The patient will require emotional support and education structured to provide him or her with essential facts. When commencing patient education it is important to determine first how much the patient already knows about diabetes and to correct any misconceptions that they may have.

The second stage requires detailed education on all aspects of diabetes (Box 10.1). Although the community nurse has her own agenda for education, it is good practice to allow the patient to determine which area he/she wishes to learn about next. Giving the patient an education 'checklist' (Box 10.1) can facilitate the patient in

---

Box 10.1   Education checklist for the patient with diabetes

- Alcohol

- British Diabetic Association

- Chiropodist
  —seen by chiropodist
  —referred to chiropodist
  —foot health education

- Contact number
  —surgery
  —community nurse
  —hospital clinic
  —diabetic nurse specialist

- Complications
  —annual MOT at surgery
  —eyes, on diagnosis and later
  —kidneys
  —feet
  —blood pressure
  —sexual health

- DSS benefits

- Diet
  —seen by dietitian
  —date to see dietitian
  —current weight and ideal body weight
  —importance of regular meals (patients with IDDM especially)

—diabetic foods
—alcohol
—special occasions
—what to do when unwell

- Driving
  —DVLA
  —insurance
  —planning a long journey
  —what to do if hypoglycaemic (not relevant if controlled by diet or a biguanide)

- Employment
  —advise to inform employer
  —shift work
  —can register disabled

- Exercise
  —benefits of exercise
  —adjusting insulin (patients with IDDM only)
  —adjusting diet

- Hypoglycaemia (patients with IDDM and those on an oral hypoglycaemic agent)
  —what causes it
  —how to recognise it
  —how to treat it
  —what happens if you don't recognise or treat it
  —telling your family and friends
  —telling employers
  —exercise
  —driving
  —nocturnal hypos
  —place of glucagon

- Hyperglycaemia
  —what causes it
  —how to recognise it
  —how to treat it
  —what happens if you don't recognise or treat it
  —when to call for help

- Identification

- Insulin (patients with IDDM only)
  —how it works

—how to inject (including mixing insulins if necessary)
—when to inject
—where to inject and rotation of sites
—storage of insulin and equipment
—disposal of equipment
—availability of equipment
—can relatives inject patient?
—never omit insulin
—what if patient forgets to inject?
—insulin dose adjustment

• Insurance
—car insurance
—life insurance

• Monitoring
—blood glucose/urinary glucose
—when to test
—recording results
—explanation of results
—goals to aim for
—urinary ketone testing (if relevant)

• Oral hypoglycaemic agents (patients with NIDDM only)
—when to take
—expected side-effects
—what to do if unwell

• Prescription exemption (not relevant if controlled by diet alone)

• Sexual Health
—contraception
—planned pregnancies and why
—HRT
—impotence

• Smoking
—advise stop

• Stress

• Travel and holidays
—long lies
—adjusting therapy

• What is diabetes?

• What to do if unwell

choosing the subject matter. Educational material must be presented in small bite-sized chunks to help the patient digest it. Reiteration, encouraging the patient to verbally reflect what has been said and reinforcement with written material all help the patient to remember.

For education to be effective, it must be continually reinforced and the patient remotivated in self-management. This is the third stage in education and this continuous cycle of education is a lifelong process.

EDUCATING THE PATIENT WITH NIDDM

For most patients with NIDDM the diagnosis of diabetes and its ensuing management commences within general practice. The community nurse is therefore ideally situated for the education of these patients.

At the first clinic visit following diagnosis the patient may well be bewildered and hence not very receptive to education (Ch. 3). However, some 'first aid' measures are appropriate until the next appointment. These would include a simple explanation of diabetes, simple adjustments made to diet following the taking of a dietary history, and the commencement of monitoring (Box 10.2). The patient should be advised regarding contact numbers should there be a problem.

As far as possible the family and friends of the patient should be included. This may not always be practical, but the patient who ushers the family out of the lounge when the community nurse visits should be discouraged from so doing.

At a further clinic visit, the patient's questions regarding diabetes would firstly be addressed. Monitoring technique would be assessed and the results discussed and explained. Since diet is the mainstay of management for the patient with NIDDM, more detailed dietary advice from the community dietitian would be appropriate.

If the patient has already commenced oral hypoglycaemic therapy it would be appropriate to advise that free prescriptions can be obtained by completing a P11 form. This is not available to patients who are treated by diet alone.

Subsequent clinic visits would include education about foot care, the benefits of clinic attendance for monitoring diabetes and the screening for complications (Box 10.2). Thereafter, all clinic visits are opportunities for reinforcing education and re-educating the patient as his/her management alters or complications develop and progress.

Box 10.2 Suggested staged approach to the education of the patient with NIDDM

- First clinic visit

  —answer patient's questions
  —simple explanation of diabetes
  —dietary history and some adjustments
  —choice of monitoring and how to undertake it
  —screening for complications, e.g. BP, neuropathy, feet, eyes, proteinuria
  —assess smoking status and offer cessation advice if necessary
  —contact numbers

- Second clinic visit

  —answer patient's questions
  —dietary reinforcement and encouragement
  —assessment of monitoring, review results
  —explanation as to what affects glucose levels
  —simple explanation of benefits of good diabetic control
  —foot health education
  —prescription exemption (if relevant)
  —DSS benefits (if relevant)
  —driving
  —related insurances
  —carry identification that the person has diabetes
  —British Diabetic Association telephone number and address

- Third clinic visit

  —answer patient's questions
  —dietary reinforcement and encouragement
  —review monitoring and explain meaning of results
  —explain the benefits of clinic attendance
  —simple explanation of diabetic complications and benefits of using the health care team to screen for these
  —benefits of exercise
  —enabling appropriate self-management during illness or any new problem

  Subsequent visits may include education regarding oral hypolgycaemic agents, travel and holidays and hypoglycaemia, if relevant

EDUCATING THE PATIENT WITH IDDM

Most patients who require insulin therapy are referred to the local hospital clinic and therefore patient education is initiated and maintained by the Diabetic Nurse Specialist (DNS). However it seems appropriate to include some aspects of patient education here as community nurses will have some responsibility for patients with IDDM.

Here too the involvement of family and friends is essential to dispel some myths about diabetes and to promote a positive approach to the patient.

The patient is usually in a state of shock at the time of diagnosis. In this particular instance, patients usually respond well to undertaking practical procedures but will not necessarily retain much factual information. Hence at the first visit, blood glucose monitoring and how to inject insulin will be taught (Box 10.3). While there may appear to be more educational material to cover with the patient on insulin, there are also more opportunities as the patient will usually be seen twice a day for a few days and thereafter followed up as necessary. Again, a staged approach is required with more detailed explanations introduced over a period of about six weeks. Since patients with IDDM tend to be seen more frequently, reinforcement of advice is easier and patients have greater opportunities to ask questions which are pertinent to them.

TOPICS WHICH REQUIRE EDUCATIONAL INPUT

Alcohol

Moderation is recommended. Alcohol taken with food seldom causes problems unless drunk to excess. When excessive alcohol is taken, hypoglycaemia can result. Onlookers may wrongly assume that the person is drunk and not appreciate that the person needs glucose.

The message therefore for the normal-weight patient is to remain within the recommended limits of 14 units of alcohol per week for women and 21 units of alcohol per week for men. Patients should be advised not to drink on an empty stomach but to consume food as well.

For those patients who are trying to follow a calorie restricted diet,

Box 10.3 Suggested staged approach to the education of the patient with IDDM

- First clinic visit
  —answer patient's questions
  —simple explanation of diabetes and the actions of insulin
  —dietary history and some adjustments
  —initiate home blood glucose monitoring
  —initiate insulin injections
  —assess smoking status and offer cessation advice if necessary
  —full medical examination
  —identification

- Within the first week
  —answer patient's questions
  —full dietary assessment and adjustments
  —how to acquire necessary equipment for injecting and monitoring
  —prescription exemption
  —DSS benefits (if relevant)
  —set goals for blood glucose levels using a staged approach
  —assessment of monitoring technique and review results
  —explanation of what affects glucose levels
  —employer
  —hypoglycaemia
  —driving
  —insurances
  —British Diabetic Association telephone number and address

- Within the second/third week
  —answer patient's questions
  —insulin dose adjustment
  —foot health education
  —alcohol
  —advantages of good diabetic control
  —the benefits of clinic attendance
  —explanation of the complications of diabetes and benefits of
    screening for diabetic complications
  —benefits and effects of exercise

- Within the first month
  —answer patient's questions
  —hyperglycaemia
  —what to do if patient is unwell

  Subsequent visits may include education regarding travel and
  holidays, sexual health matters, stress related problems

specific guidance is required and they should be referred to the dietician for this (Ch. 6).

It is difficult to manage diabetes if the patient concerned has problems with excessive alcohol intake. Metformin is contraindicated in liver disease and both sulphonylureas and insulin can cause profound hypoglycaemia in the presence of excess alcohol. Under these circumstances, loosening of diabetic control is necessary. The patient should be encouraged to eat while drinking and to consume some food prior to retiring in the evening.

Benefits

As mentioned earlier, those patients whose diabetes is controlled by the use of oral hypoglycaemic agents or insulin are eligible for prescription exemption. Previously patients controlled by diet were also exempt but this is no longer the case as the 'diabetic diet' is now regarded as healthy eating and not a 'special diet'. To apply for prescription exemption, the patient must complete a P11 form which is available from the local Social Security office, some GP surgeries and local pharmacists. The patient's GP, who is required to complete part of the form, will then send it to the Family Health Services Authority (FHSA). The FHSA issue the exemption certificate and on its presentation, the patient has exemption from paying for any items which are available on prescription. Prescription exemption can make a financial saving for those patients who have multiple pathology requiring several different medications.

There are other benefits to which people with diabetes may be entitled. Further advice may be obtained by contacting the local Citizens' Advice Bureau, the Welfare Rights Adviser or Social Services Department. While there are several Social Security benefits available, not all people with diabetes are eligible for them (Balance 1995). All people with diabetes are eligible for a free NHS eye test. However, only those on a low income are eligible for NHS vouchers for glasses.

British Diabetic Association (BDA)

The BDA is a charitable organisation, set up in 1934 by Dr R D Lawrence and the author H G Wells, both of whom had diabetes. Through its many committees and functions, the BDA promotes care for people with diabetes in both education and research.

Under the auspices of the BDA there are over 400 local branches and groups which are run entirely by volunteers. These branches and groups offer support and companionship to people with diabetes and their carers. In 1994, the first of several proposed regional offices was opened in Glasgow, Scotland to promote the work of the BDA at a regional level.

Joining the BDA affords the free issue of the 'Balance' magazine bimonthly and information on local BDA branches. The 'Balance' magazine is a patients' magazine and is a rich resource on current issues in diabetes management. Self-help groups play an important part in caring for people with diabetes and patients should be encouraged to link up with their local group.

For the health care professional, the BDA is a valuable resource centre which offers help and advice on a wide variety of topics. Health care professionals also have the opportunity to join professional sections of the BDA which offer the possibility of attending conferences and receiving professional journals.

Driving

Until recently, all people with diabetes who drove were legally obliged to inform the Driver and Vehicle Licensing Authority (DVLA) and their own insurance company that they had diabetes. Regulations have recently been altered and now only patients on oral agents or insulin therapy are required to inform the DVLA. The responsibility for informing the DVLA lies with the patient. The primary health care team must ensure that the patient is aware of this obligation.

The DVLA, however, would still like all people with diabetes to notify them of their diabetes because it has an obligation to remind all people with the condition that they must inform the DVLA should visual complications occur (Roland 1992).

Once the DVLA has been informed that the patient has diabetes, a driving licence is issued which is only valid for 1–3 years. It is renewed after that time for a further 1–3 years provided there is a satisfactory medical report. Once the person reaches 70 years of age it is renewed annually subject to a satisfactory medical report. This report is usually obtained from the general practitioner or hospital consultant.

The situation is currently different in Northern Ireland. The regulations state that every diabetic patient must inform the Driver and Vehicle Licensing authority for Northern Ireland, regardless of their treatment. It is anticipated that this will change in the near future and will be brought into line with the DVLA. Those patients who are controlled by diet or diet and tablets are issued with a licence for 10 years. Those patients requiring insulin are issued with a licence for 1–3 years (Deegan 1995a).

The greatest risk to the patient and others is of hypoglycaemia while driving. For this reason, patients who are taking a sulphonylurea or insulin are usually prohibited from driving any form of public service transport or heavy goods vehicle.

It is currently against the law for a Large Goods Vehicle licence (LGV) or a Passenger Carrying Vehicle licence to be issued to a patient requiring insulin therapy. However, for some patients with IDDM an LGV licence may be granted on a discretionary basis (Frier 1991). As the UK becomes more involved in the European Union, this discretionary basis is likely to disappear.

For those patients who are on a sulphonylurea or insulin the prevention of hypoglycaemia is paramount. Glucose must be kept in the car within easy access. If the patient should feel hypoglycaemic, they must be advised to stop the car (using the hard shoulder on a motorway), switch off the engine, get out of the driver's seat and take glucose to correct the hypoglycaemia. All this is required because the patient could legally be charged with being in control of a vehicle while under the influence of drugs (Frier 1991). The patient should not recommence the journey until fully recovered from hypoglycaemia.

Long journeys must be planned to allow frequent stops for food and rest and to monitor blood glucose levels. A journey should not be undertaken when the patient has injected insulin without having eaten.

All diabetic drivers should be advised to have their eyesight checked regularly and not to drive if their vision deteriorates suddenly or if their visual acuity with glasses is less than 6/12 in both eyes. Any eyesight changes must be notified to the DVLA.

While most citizens enjoy the pleasures of car driving, for the patient with diabetes this is one aspect of their lifestyle which requires regular review and which with progression of diabetic complications may be denied them.

Employment

Patients who are in employment are strongly advised to inform their employer of their diabetes. For those patients who have NIDDM

Box 10.4   Occupations which are prohibited to patients with IDDM

- airline pilot
- train driver
- armed forces
- police force

- prison service
- fire brigade
- merchant navy

---

there is not usually any problem with this. Patients who have IDDM may find that certain aspects of their job are restricted because of the risk of hypoglycaemia.

There are however some forms of employment which are prohibited to any patient who has IDDM (Box 10.4). The BDA are currently working hard to reduce this 'blanket ban' on recruitment and are pressing for individual assessment (Deegan 1995b). Any employment where hypoglycaemia may not only endanger the life of the patient but also the lives of others is prohibited. Those patients who are currently employed within those spheres and who then acquire IDDM may be allowed to continue in employment but in a less demanding post. There are other forms of employment which may be considered as inadvisable for a patient with IDDM to pursue, again because of the risk of hypoglycaemia (Box 10.5).

While it is not impossible for patients with IDDM to undertake shift work, they will need advice regarding insulin doses and the balancing of food intake to accommodate this. Where this is relevant, the patient would be advised to visit their DNS for detailed, personal advice.

Time off to attend clinics should be negotiated with the person's employer. On average, people with diabetes do have a slightly higher sickness rate than nondiabetics but they compensate for this by their generally good performance records (Greene & Geroy 1993).

Box 10.5   Type of occupation which would be inadvisable for patients with IDDM

deep-sea diver
steeplejack
blast furnaceman

Diabetes is a disease for which a person can register as disabled. Patients should be warned of the employment consequences of being thus labelled. They should also be advised that, once registered as disabled, they cannot request removal from the register at a later date.

Exercise

Exercise is good for everyone. Apart from promoting a feeling of well-being, it improves the tissue sensitivity to insulin. As the patient with NIDDM tends to be older, so the recommended form of exercise would be to build on what they currently do rather than commence some new strenuous form of exercise. An example of this would be to alight from the bus a stop early and walk the remaining distance rather than start jogging for 15 minutes each day. However, for those patients with NIDDM who wish to pursue a new form of exercise, a full medical examination by their general practitioner is advisable to ensure that there are no contraindications. For the older patient, warm-up and cool-down exercises are essential. The patient with NIDDM who is taking a sulphonylurea is at risk of hypoglycaemia. Home blood glucose monitoring and consuming extra carbohydrates are essential to prevent, detect and treat hypoglycaemia. Those patients concerned should be advised on an individual basis. Daily exercise is beneficial but few people seem able or willing to adjust their lifestyle to take account of this.

For the patient with IDDM, exercise can induce hypoglycaemia. There are two ways by which the patient can prevent this occurring. If the exercise is planned in advance, the patient can reduce the relevant insulin (Ch. 5) by a certain amount and/or consume extra carbohydrate before and hourly during the exercise.

The reduction in insulin dose will be discussed with the DNS beforehand. To do this effectively, the patient must be sufficiently motivated to undertake HBGM prior to exercise, immediately afterwards and for several hours thereafter. On the basis of these results and by a system of trial and error, patients can learn by how much their insulin should be altered in response to differing amounts of exercise. This takes a tremendous amount of commitment from the patient and not all are willing to follow this regime strictly.

In addition to insulin dose adjustment, the patient is advised to consume about 20–40 g of extra carbohydrate before and hourly during exercise (Ch. 6). An example of this would be 400 ml of milk and two digestive biscuits prior to exercise followed hourly by a mini-size Mars bar or four squares of chocolate for the duration of the exercise.

The prevention of hypoglycaemia which is exercise-induced partly depends on the type of exercise, its frequency and intensity. People's perception of what is exercise varies markedly. The person who frequently walks with children to school may be very active and does not consider this as exercise while the person who works out on an exercise bike at home for ten minutes regards him/herself as taking exercise. It is important to determine each individual person's normal lifestyle so that advice can be appropriate.

It should also be remembered that exercise has a hypoglycaemic effect for several hours after the exercise has ceased. Hence the patient who goes swimming is unlikely to become hypoglycaemic in the pool but is more likely to feel hypoglycaemic a few hours later.

The intensity of the exercise will affect the rate at which hypoglycaemia develops. Thus a gentle walk along a forest path may gradually reduce the blood sugar level resulting in hypoglycaemia several hours later, whereas half an hour on a squash court will rapidly reduce a blood glucose level and so hypoglycaemia will be more obvious sooner.

Patients should be guided and advised regarding their own requirements on an individual basis and it is impossible to give any further prescriptive care.

Case Study 10.1

A female patient in her later 30s, who has IDDM, complains of frequent hypoglycaemic episodes which she cannot explain. She had been asked to keep a detailed diary of these episodes in relation to her insulin doses, exercise and food. On close examination of her diary it appears that she is always hypoglycaemic on a Thursday and a Saturday in the late evening.

In discussion with the patient it transpires that she goes to an aerobics class immediately after work each Thursday and on a Saturday afternoon. On a Thursday she does not take her insulin until after the class and then has her usual evening meal. On a Saturday, she takes 20 g extra carbohydrate prior to the class and has a few alcoholic drinks with friends afterwards.

The woman would be advised to reduce her Thursday morning insulin by a small amount (given that the exercise occurs late in the afternoon) and to consume 20 g of carbohydrate prior to her aerobics class. With regard to a Saturday, she could safely reduce her morning insulin by a greater amount than on Thursday and, when socialising after the class, consume extra carbohydrates to offset the effects of the alcohol.

It should be emphasised that these adjustments are made only when the patient is undertaking strenuous exercise. Should she decide not to attend her aerobics class, the normal dose of insulin would be taken.

Further consultation showed that the patient was no longer experiencing hypoglycaemic episodes, her blood glucose levels were as consistent as before and the patient felt more confident about adjusting her insulin and diet to accommodate exercise.

Hyperglycaemia

This is the main prevailing clinical sign when a person is diagnosed as having diabetes. As described earlier, it causes the clinical symptoms of polyuria and polydipsia. Recurrence of these symptoms, following the introduction of successful treatment, indicates a deterioration in metabolic control (Box 10.6). Patients should be alerted to this fact and be advised to seek help under these circumstances (McDowell 1991). Hyperglycaemia builds up over days and may be due to any one of several factors (Box 10.7). Patients can be reassured that they have time on their side to seek advice.

Box 10.6 Signs and symptoms of hyperglycaemia	
polyuria	hypotension
polydipsia	hypovolaemia
glycosuria	tachycardia
dehydration	abdominal pain
weight loss	cold, dry skin
general tiredness	acidotic breath
blurring of vision	deep rapid breathing
itching and skin infections	confusion and restlessness
pain and paraesthesia	coma
in feet and limbs	death
nausea and vomiting	

Box 10.7 Factors that affect blood glucose levels	
Hyperglycaemia	Hypoglycaemia
• not enough insulin	• too much insulin
• not enough exercise	• exercise which patient not used to
• too much food	• not enough food, delaying or missing a meal
• any other illness	• recovering from an illness
• stress	• alcohol
• erratic absorption of insulin	• erratic absorption of insulin
• other medication	

Left untreated, the metabolic decompensation might progress to non-ketotic hyperosmolar coma in the older patient with NIDDM or ketoacidosis in the patient requiring insulin (Ch. 1; Box 10.6). Both are life-threatening conditions and it is essential that the patient seeks help sooner rather than later.

The treatment of hyperglycaemia largely depends on its severity. For some patients the introduction of an oral hypoglycaemia agent may be all that is required. For others, hospital admission is essential for insulin therapy and rehydration. After such an episode, the cause should be established and, if possible, the patient advised how to prevent it in the future.

Hypoglycaemia

Education about hypoglycaemia features prominently in caring for patients with diabetes. Patients are frightened of hypoglycaemia and so may deliberately keep their blood glucose levels high. While this is understandable, patients must be taught how to achieve healthy glucose profiles and prevent, recognise and treat hypoglycaemia.

Those patients who take a sulphonylurea or insulin are at risk of hypoglycaemia. In the elderly, hypoglycaemia may simulate a transient ischaemic attack or a cerebral vascular accident. It is therefore important to check a blood glucose level in any elderly patient who presents with neurological signs. Although these may appear to be of a minor nature, all such patients should be admitted to hospital for 24 hours for observation.

The onset of hypoglycaemia is usually rapid and the patient is required to recognise and treat the early symptoms immediately (the 'warning signs'). The signs and symptoms are listed in Box 8.3, page 177. Abnormal lowering of blood glucose causes stimulation of the sympathetic nervous system and then progressive depression of brain function.

Stimulating the sympathetic nervous system causes a release of adrenaline which results in the clinical signs and symptoms of pallor, sweating and tachycardia. As glucose is essential to maintain normal metabolism within brain cells, so severe and prolonged hypoglycaemia results in a gradual deterioration in brain function. Patients may experience symptoms of numbness or paraesthesia, dizziness and lightheadedness, altered behaviour and deterioration in conscious level until coma develops.

Treatment of hypoglycaemia

Each patient has warning signs of impending hypoglycaemia which are specific to the individual. For some patients it will be a feeling of faintness, for others it may be tingling around the lips. It is necessary for patients to appreciate that one symptom is adequate warning of hypoglycaemia and action must be taken. Patients are encouraged to discover their own specific warning sign. When this is recognised, the patient can take about 10–20 g carbohydrate in the form of glucose tablets and should 'feel better' within 10–15 minutes.

Some of the other symptoms will occur if the patient does not recognise hypoglycaemia or chooses to ignore the warning sign. At this stage, the patient may need assistance to take oral glucose in the form of a liquid. An example would be Lucozade or similar (ensuring that it is not of a 'diet' variety). Glucose in the form of a viscous gel ('Hypostop') can be squeezed into the mouth and is of particular value in children. Its use in adults is not recommended by some clinicians because of the danger of aspiration (MacCuish 1993).

Once the patient has come round from the hypoglycaemic episode, extra carbohydrate of a more solid form should be consumed. The lower the patient's blood glucose level the longer it will take for the patient to 'feel well' afterwards. The patient may feel quite groggy and mentally slow for a few hours after the event.

Patients who have a hypoglycaemic episode during the night usually miss the warning signs because of sleep and are therefore at risk of a more severe attack. A nocturnal hypoglycaemic episode is frightening for the patient and the patient's bedfellow! Those patients who require reassurance about this are advised to check their blood glucose level before retiring at night and, if low, to consume extra carbohydrate before sleeping.

Left untreated, the patient would eventually lapse into a hypo-glycaemic coma which requires assistance from someone else to treat it. Relatives and friends can be taught how to administer glucagon 1 mg intramuscularly. Glucagon is available in convenient packs containing 1 mg of the dried form of the agent and 1 ml diluting solution. In this form the hormone is stable for at least 2 years when stored at room temperature. The patient and family should be advised to check the expiry date regularly and obtain another prescription prior to the current vial expiring.

Glucagon can be rapidly dissolved and injected subcutaneously, intramuscularly or intravenously and should restore consciousness within 10–20 minutes. The patient should then be encouraged to con-sume at least 30 g oral carbohydrate in order to replace glucose stores.

One problem with glucagon is that it causes nausea and vomiting, so although the patient becomes more responsive, he/she may refuse to eat or drink. It then becomes a battle of wills! It is necessary for the patient to eat to replenish liver glycogen stores and prevent secondary hypoglycaemia developing. However, the patient may resist.

Glucagon is less effective when the patient has been unconscious for a prolonged period of time (MacCuish et al 1970). Under these circumstances, an intravenous injection of 50% dextrose is preferred and this is usually carried out in the hospital Accident and Emergency Department.

Patients usually experience a severe headache for up to 24 hours after a prolonged episode of hypoglycaemia.

Aftercare from a hypoglycaemic episode

Patients should be advised not to test their blood glucose level for up to 24 hours after a hypoglycaemic episode unless they feel hypo-glycaemic again. Hypoglycaemia causes the body to mobilise stored glucose reserves which, with the treatment of the hypoglycaemia, may cause a temporary hyperglycaemia.

The patient should seek advice following any severe hypoglycaemic episode or any episode which he or she cannot explain.

It is now known that maintaining blood glucose levels as near normal as possible carries with it a threefold increased risk of hypoglycaemia (DCCT Research Group 1993). It is also recognised that one hypoglycaemic episode hinders a non-diabetic person from recognising another episode if it occurs a few hours later, which may have a bearing on the patient with IDDM (Heller & Cryer 1991). There are also some patients who get no warning sign, or lose their warning sign, of impending hypoglycaemia (Frier 1993).

Loosening of diabetic control is the only option available for those patients who have no warning sign of hypoglycaemia, have had unexplained severe hypoglycaemia or who are unable to correct hypoglycaemia for whatever reason.

Patient education is vital in recognising and treating hypoglycaemia (McDowell 1991). Friends and relatives should be actively encouraged to participate in the same.

Identification

All patients are advised to carry some form of identification to inform others that they have diabetes. This may be a card, an alert medic bracelet or similar locket. Most pharmaceutical companies produce identification cards and there are advertisements in the Balance magazine for these products.

Insurance

Patients should be advised to inform all the insurance companies from which they have relevant policies once they are diagnosed as having diabetes. The responsibility for informing the various companies lies with the patient. This includes driving insurance. Failure to do so may jeopardise future claims. Some companies confer an additional premium for diabetics. It is therefore important to shop around and receive quotations from several different companies. The BDA have special arrangements with various insurance companies for people with diabetes. Advice can be given on motor insurance, life assurance and travel insurance. Contact the BDA for further information.

Sexual health

Females

For some women who are insulin-dependent, there may be an alteration in insulin requirement around the time of menstruation (Steel 1991a). Some women find that they require to increase the insulin dose for a few days while others need to decrease the dose. Each woman has to be considered individually.

Women with good diabetic control have similar fertility to non-diabetic women. Hence it is important that contraceptive advice is offered.

All forms of contraception currently available can be used by women with diabetes. However they are not all equally suitable. The combined oral contraceptive pill is acceptable if restricted in use to short periods of time and to young women without diabetic complications or risk factors (Steel 1991b). The progesterone-only pill therefore has a wider scope for use. Mechanical devices—intrauterine devices, caps and sheaths—have a fairly high failure rate, unless they are used very carefully, within the population as a whole. They are therefore not recommended where pregnancy is contraindicated. The intrauterine device has the potential to cause increased infection in women with diabetes and so is not favoured. Sterilisation is a suitable method of contraception for both male and female patients with diabetes once they are sure that their families are completed.

Planning for pregnancy is of vital importance. Women with poorly controlled diabetes have reduced fertility. However, any woman may become pregnant whether her diabetes is well controlled or not. Poor diabetic control at the time of conception is associated with an increased risk of fetal malformation (Lowy 1991). It is therefore important that all women of childbearing age are made aware of this fact and encouraged to achieve optimal diabetic control before stopping contraception. The majority of women of child-bearing age with diabetes will be insulin-dependent. However a small number may be on oral hypoglycaemic agents. These drugs must be replaced by insulin prior to conception.

Hormone replacement therapy (HRT) for women with diabetes might have positive effects as a means of reducing coronary mortality. Each woman requesting HRT should be assessed individually. It is unlikely that a woman would be refused HRT provided there were no contraindications (Selby & Oakley 1992).

Males

Impotence is usually under-reported by patients with diabetes. It is due to neurological and arterial components and is usually irreversible (Ch. 8). Impotence which is due to psychogenic causes may respond to expert counselling. Male patients should be informed of this potential complication and encouraged to report if it is present and causing problems. The possibility of impotence resulting from poorly controlled diabetes should serve as a good motivating factor to maintaining good diabetic control!

Smoking

The combination of smoking and diabetes is a serious matter. As both smoking and diabetes predispose towards an increased risk of coronary heart disease and arterial disease, so the patient who smokes is at greater risk of having a heart attack, a cerebrovascular accident or developing peripheral vascular disease. Patients may not be aware of the increased risks due to both conditions and every effort must be made strongly to encourage patients who smoke to stop.

Those patients wishing to stop should be referred to the smoking cessation clinic in the practice. There are various methods recommended to help people stop smoking. These include the use of nicotine patches, group or individual counselling and hypnosis.

Stress

Stress, both physical and mental, can have adverse effects on a patient's blood glucose levels. It is important that poor diabetic control is not always attributed to poor compliance with diabetic therapy but other aspects of the patient's life are also explored. This holistic approach to care views the patient as a whole person and not just the sum of the parts. The reader is referred to Chapter 3 on adopting a counselling approach for patients.

Travel and holidays

Prior to foreign travel, the patient must receive adequate immunisations for the country that they plan to visit. They should also ensure they have adequate medical insurance for their travel.

Carrying identification that the person has diabetes can prevent awkward situations at Customs if needles and syringes are detected in baggage. This may take the form of a medic alert bracelet or a letter from the patient's GP or hospital consultant.

When travelling west, extra hours in a day do not usually require extra doses of oral hypoglycaemic agents. In a greatly shortened day, when travelling from west to east, one dose of hypoglycaemic agent may be safely omitted. Patients on insulin therapy should receive advice from the DNS regarding insulin doses to accommodate time changes and variable eating times while travelling.

All patients should take an ample supply of their medications and monitoring equipment with them. It is advisable that they keep a portion as hand luggage and distribute the rest throughout their baggage so that if one bag should go missing, they will still have a supply of the necessary equipment remaining. Insulin should not go into luggage in the hold of the aircraft as there is the risk of the insulin freezing at high altitudes. As an additional safeguard, the traveller's companion may carry spare insulin.

Insulin does not denature very easily and can be maintained at 25 degrees centigrade for several months with only a small loss of potency (Steel 1991c). However, to prevent excessive temperature changes, patients should be taught to transport their insulin at refrigeration temperatures using a cool bag. On arrival at their destination, patients are encouraged to store their insulin in a hotel refrigerator and to keep a spare supply safely in a cool bag in their room, away from direct sunlight. It is good practice always to check each vial of insulin visually prior to using it, to ensure that the vial has its normal appearance.

The BDA have various booklets for the traveller regarding the availability of oral hypoglycaemic agents and insulins in other countries, food and drink, health agreements and useful phrases for the most commonly visited European countries.

While on holiday, patients with IDDM can have an occasional long lie in bed! It is probably advisable that they take their insulin and breakfast at the usual time before retiring for an extra sleep. For those who find this unacceptable, the occasional later injection of insulin will probably not do much harm although the patient would be advised to delay the evening dose of insulin to accommodate the morning delay.

Holiday activities may involve strenuous exercise. What should happen to insulin doses and carbohydrate intake? While extra exercise may require less insulin, it is not usually a problem to eat more when on holiday. Hence, by maintaining the patient's current insulin dose, extra exercise is usually accommodated by consuming more food and so avoiding hypoglycaemia.

Sunbathing on a beach may, for some people, be considered hard work but for most people is less strenuous than a normal day's activities! However, as sunbathing causes skin temperature to rise, there may be increased absorption of insulin which can cause hypo-glycaemia. Patients should therefore be advised to keep glucose readily available even while sunbathing.

What to do if unwell

The most important advice to be given here is to seek help and to seek it quickly (Box 10.8). Patients who are unwell are usually off their food. When unable to eat, patients tend to stop their drugs or insulin therapy, and metabolic control can be rapidly lost under those circumstances.

For the patient who is controlled by diet alone or diet and a small dose of oral agent, this may not pose a great problem. The chances are that these patients are overweight anyway and so a few days of reduced appetite may in fact be very beneficial! Should their illness be prolonged then it would be necessary to monitor their blood glucose levels and urinary ketones at least twice a day.

Box 10.8   What to do if unwell

- Seek help quickly.
- Never stop taking medication or insulin.
- If unable to eat food, take small, frequent amounts of semi-solids. Examples of 10 g of carbohydrate which could be taken are:
  50 g scoop ice cream
  200 ml milk
  200 ml tomato soup
  50 ml Lucozade
  half a small carton of fruit yoghurt.
- Drink about three litres of water or sugar free fluids per day to prevent dehydration.
- Increase self-monitoring to twice a day if urine testing and four times a day if blood testing.
- If facilities are available, test urine for ketones if there is a 2% glycosuria or if blood glucose levels are above 15 mmol/l.
- Contact the GP if any of the following apply:
  the presence of ketonuria
  vomiting
  abdominal pain
  elevated temperature
  illness that lasts longer than 24 hours.

Patients taking larger doses of metformin (above 500 mg twice a day) should continue with treatment. As this drug does not cause hypoglycaemia there are no great risks of the glucose level dropping too low. In the severely ill patient, there is however a risk of lactic acidosis occurring.

Those patients who are taking larger doses of a sulphonylurea (e.g. Gliclazide above 80 mg) will still require to continue them. Since the sulphonylureas can cause hypoglycaemia, patients must replace the normal carbohydrate content of their diet with food or drink. Monitoring of blood glucose levels is essential at least four times a day and urinary ketone testing at least twice a day. Advice must be sought if there are any elevated blood glucose levels and any ketonuria.

Patients with IDDM must never stop taking their insulin. During an illness, they may require increased amounts of insulin; even when the patient is not eating as normal. Carbohydrates must be replaced with palatable foods or fluids (Ch. 6). HBGM should be increased to at least four times a day and urinary testing for ketones commenced four times a day.

All these measures are to detect deteriorating diabetic control when a patient feels unwell. The patient should also be advised to seek help from the health care team especially if there is any indication that his or her condition is deteriorating. In this instance, the patient should be referred to the diabetic consultant as soon as possible and hospital admission may be required.

SUMMARY

Effective patient education is time-consuming and its effects are difficult to measure on an individual patient's lifestyle and quality of life. While education is central to all diabetic care, the rights of the patient either to refuse the education or to alter their lifestyle in response to the education must be considered.

To assist patients coping with diabetes and the necessary lifestyle changes that may be involved, educational material must be readable, understandable and relevant to the individual person. Educational sessions must be paced and presented to suit the individual person's learning style. While health care professionals have their own agenda for these educational sessions, to make them more effective the content should be decided by the patient concerned.

To determine if the educational programme is effective or not, it is essential to audit the educational achievement.

REFERENCES

Balance Magazine 1995 Getting the benefit. Balance 145:14–16
The DCCT Research Group 1993 The effect of intensive treatment of diabetes on the development and progression of long term complications in insulin-dependent diabetes mellitus. New England Journal of Medicine 14:329:977–986
Deegan G 1995a Medical Q and As. Balance 144:36
Deegan G 1995b Medical Q and As. Balance 145:44
Frier B M 1991 Driving and diabetes mellitus. In: Pickup J C, Williams G (eds) 1991 Textbook of diabetes. Blackwell Scientific, Oxford
Frier B M 1993 Hypoglycaemia unawareness. In: Frier B M, Fisher B M (eds) 1993 Hypoglycaemia and diabetes. Edward Arnold, London
Greene D, Geroy G D 1993 Diabetes and job performance: an empirical investigation. The Diabetes Educator 19: 4:293–298
Heller S R, Cryer P E 1991 Reduced neuroendocrine and symptomatic responses to subsequent hypoglycaemia after one episode of hypoglycaemia in nondiabetic humans. Diabetes 40:223–226
Lowy C 1991 Pregnancy and diabetes. In: Pickup J C, Williams G (eds) 1991 Textbook of diabetes. Blackwell Scientific, Oxford
MacCuish A C 1993 Treatment of hypoglycaemia. In: Frier B M, Fisher B M (eds) 1993 Hypoglycaemia and diabetes. Edward Arnold, London
MacCuish A C, Munro J F, Duncan L J P 1970 Treatment of hypoglycaemic coma with glucagon, intravenous dextrose and mannitol infusion in a hundred diabetics. Lancet ii:946–949
McDowell J R S 1991 Prevention is better than coma. Professional Nurse 7:3:150–156
Overland J E, Hoskins P L, McGill M J, Yue D K 1993 Low literacy: a problem in diabetes education. Diabetic Medicine 10:847–850
Petterson T, Dornan T L, Albert T, Lee P 1994 Are information leaflets given to elderly people with diabetes easy to read? Diabetic Medicine 11:111–113
Roland J (ed) 1992 (Winter) Diabetes update. British Diabetic Association, London
Selby P L, Oakley C E 1992 Women's problems and diabetes. Innovative care. Diabetic Medicine 9:3:290–292
Steel J M 1991a Sexual function in diabetic women. In: Pickup J C, Williams G (eds) 1991 Textbook of diabetes. Blackwell Scientific, Oxford
Steel J M 1991b Contraception for diabetic women. In: Pickup J C, Williams G (eds) 1991 Textbook of diabetes. Blackwell Scientific, Oxford
Steel J M 1991c Travel and diabetes mellitus. In: Pickup J C, Williams G (eds) 1991 Textbook of diabetes. Blackwell Scientific, Oxford

Auditing standards of care

Frank Sullivan

■ CONTENTS

INTRODUCTION

Ever tried. Ever failed.
No Matter.
Try again, fail again. Fail better.
          Samuel Beckett

In each of the previous chapters readers have learnt how to deliver high quality care for diabetic patients within the community setting. This chapter discusses the need to assess and monitor performance, and how this should be done to improve performance.

WHY AUDIT PRACTICE?

We know that those general practices which involve community nurses in the care of diabetic patients achieve better results than those who do not (Table 11.1). However we also know from our daily work that there are still areas of care which could be improved. These everyday

Table 11.1 Differences in diabetic care when a practice nurse is involved (Reproduced with kind permission from Stearn and Sullivan 1993)

		Nurse not involved	Nurse involved
Number of practices		28	22
Structure (number of practices using these features in the last year)	Flow sheet	2	14*
	Snellen chart	18	21*
Process (items recorded in practice in the last year)	Unknown smoking status	50%	40% (-0.2–21.7)
	Blood pressure	75%	82% (8.9 – 34.0)**
	Weight	23%	45% (1.2 – 13.9)**
	Feet	6%	28% (9.7 – 33.2)
	Visual acuity	2%	13% (3.0 – 19.6)**
Outcome	Mean HbA$_{1c}$	11%	10.5% (−0.8 – 0.2)**
	Admitted during last 12 months	14.8%	13.7% (−4.3 – 3.3)

* P< 0.05 chi-squared; **P > 0.05 analysis of variance.

impressions are borne out by research evidence which suggests that despite our best efforts to deliver high quality care we often fail to diagnose and treat appropriately all our patients with chronic diseases such as diabetes (Stearn & Sullivan 1993). Audit therefore defines and monitors the quality of care which we provide. It clarifies the activities pursued and the resources necessary for so doing. Through audit, shortcomings can be identified and more resources justified. It provides an objective evaluation of a 'gut feeling' and it also ensures that safety levels are being met. Hence there are obvious benefits in ensuring the best use of resources to provide good quality patient care.

Audit is the process by which current practice is evaluated, and is usually thought of as a cyclical process (Figure 11.1). To be effective the cycle needs to be repeated to see whether the changes implemented have improved care. It has been shown to produce improvements in diabetic care towards the levels of excellence to which we all aspire. Rather than simply going round in circles, the purpose of audit is to progress. So perhaps an image of a gradually ascending spiral is more appropriate than a circle. Thus audit is simply one

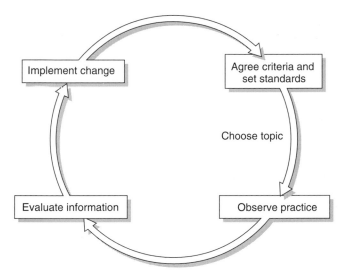

Fig. 11.1 The audit cycle.

way of discovering whether you are doing what you ought to be doing and, if not, how to make improvements.

Within the UK, the government has recognised the value of audit and has provided a financial incentive to general practices: in order to claim a 'chronic disease management payment' for care of diabetic patients, practices must audit the care provided (Kemple & Hayter 1991).

The format of this chapter is first to get the jargon out of the way. Thereafter questions will be answered which arise from applying the audit cycle to diabetes (Box 11.1, page 239). The answers to these questions will set diabetic care within the wider context of standard setting and give guidelines for community nurses working in general practice (Sullivan & Stearn 1992). So first let's get those basic definitions settled.

JARGON USED IN AUDIT

Audit

Audit is 'the systematic and critical analysis of the quality of clinical care. This includes the procedures used for diagnosis and treatment, the associated use of resources and the effect of care on the outcome and quality of life for the patient' (Working for Patients 1989).

Standards

Standards are the level of care which must be reached in order to achieve the desired clinical outcomes. These should be derived from current clinical knowledge. However it is important that standards which have been set are realistic and capable of being achieved.

Bearing in mind the difficulties of ensuring adequate recording and respect for patients' rights, it would be realistic to set a standard as follows: '80% of diabetic women between the ages of 16 and 40 should have pre-pregnancy counselling recorded in their GP notes.'

In contrast, given the seriousness of diabetic eye disease, a more rigorous standard should be set, for example: '100% of diabetic patients should have an annual eye check (visual acuity and fundoscopy) by a competent person.'

Standards therefore describe the professionally agreed level at which you want things to happen appropriate to the population addressed. They should encapsulate a definition of 'good practice'. A standard must not only be achievable but also desirable, observable and measurable (Kendall & Kitson 1986).

Criteria

Criteria are statements about the delivery of care which can be translated into measurement in order to assess quality. In other words, it is a measure by which the quality of care can be judged. Take for example the standard for successful pregnancy outcome in women with diabetes. One criterion for this would be the recording of pre-pregnancy counselling in the notes of women.

Criteria therefore describe in detail what is required in clinical practice in order to achieve the desired standard. They should be derived by professional consensus and should therefore be widely recognised as being important, worthwhile and clinically sound. Criteria cover all aspects of care and can be subdivided into different categories.

Structure criteria

These describe the facilities and staff resources which must be provided in order to achieve the standard required. It covers aspects such as buildings, equipment, paramedical and laboratory services, training of staff and agreed procedures or policies. Examples include:

- A room which can be suitably darkened for eye examination is available within the practice.

- The practice has appropriate and well-maintained equipment.
- The community nurse has received education at appropriate nationally approved courses.
- The practice has a register of all patients with diabetes.
- The practice has a protocol for shared care with the local diabetic specialists.

Process criteria

These describe which actions must take place in order to achieve the standard. These would include assessment of the delivery of care as well as the techniques and resources used. Process criteria also include evaluation of the competence of staff carrying out the task. For example:

- The practice operates an effective review system.
- The community nurse assesses the patients' understanding and knowledge of diabetes.
- Dietary advice is given as required.
- Patients with diabetes are taught self-monitoring techniques when appropriate.

Outcome criteria

The outcome of care is dependent upon adequate structures and processes being in place. Outcome criteria therefore measure the final result of the care process.

- The patient is able to carry out self-monitoring.
- The patient's glycated haemoglobin results improve.
- The number of patients admitted to hospital with hypoglycaemia is reduced.
- There is a reduction in reported complications over a given period of time.
- The patient states that diabetes does not interfere with his/her lifestyle.

An example of a set standard with appropriate criteria is to be found in Table 11.2.

Guidelines

Guidelines are 'Systematically developed statements to assist practitioner and patient decisions about appropriate health care for speci-

Table 11.2   Standard: All patients with non-insulin-dependent diabetes mellitus will be given the opportunity to receive an annual 'MOT'

Structure	Process	Outcome
Active register recall system	Receptionist identifies and recalls relevant patients	Patient receives reminder and attends clinic
Clinic time allocated	Nurse sets up mini-clinic	Patient has designated time
Facilities for eye testing	Nurse checks visual acuity and instills eye drops GP examines back of the eyes	Patient's visual acuity and back of eyes are checked
Equipment for screening tests	Nurse checks weight, assesses feet, sensation Nurse removes blood for analysis	Patient reassured Patient has blood checked

fic clinical circumstances' (Field & Lohr 1990). Guidelines are therefore a set of recommendations for medical and nursing staff on how the patients should be cared for. Examples are:

- Patients should undergo annual screening for diabetic complications.
- Optic fundi should be examined through dilated pupils.
- Levels of blood pressure are defined at which treatment should be instigated.

Protocols

Protocols are 'The detailed development of the broad principles in a guideline amended for local application' (CRAG 1993). Take for example a general practice where the GP has little experience in examining the eyes of patients with diabetes. Although the Health Board guidelines may state that patients should be referred to an ophthalmologist when they have preproliferative retinopathy, this may be inappropriate in this case due to the lack of experience of the GP. Therefore a local protocol may be established recommending that all patients showing only background retinopathy will be referred to the ophthalmologist for annual eye screening. This is due to the fact that

---

Box 11.1   Questions which arise from applying the audit cycle to diabetic care

- How should we decide which aspects of diabetic care to audit?
- Which criteria should we use to investigate a topic?
- How do we set standards that are relevant in our day-to-day work?
- How can we compare our performance with those standards?
- How does demonstrating deficiencies help to produce improvements?
- Is it all worthwhile?

---

the features of background retinopathy are easily recognised, even by the inexperienced GP.

Now that the jargon is out of the way let us consider the questions which arise from applying the audit cycle to diabetic care (Box 11.1).

HOW SHOULD WE DECIDE WHICH ASPECTS OF DIABETIC CARE TO AUDIT?

Case Study 11.1

The local Health Centre is a 7500-patient, 4-partner training practice with two part time practice nurses, two district nurses, two health visitors and a bathing attendant in an inner city area of Central Scotland. In the past they have been involved in only a few trainee and undergraduate audit projects, but spurred on by the new Chronic Disease Management regulations they decide to audit diabetic care for the 63 known diabetic patients on their list. They decide to focus on the areas of registration, recall and regular eye checks (the 3 Rs).

In this instance, the Health Centre practice has chosen to audit firstly those topics which they consider to be of highest priority and which are fundamental for the running of the diabetic clinic. However, readers may define a different set of priorities for their own practice. Alternatively, they may choose to audit a topic which is an area of concern, usually because of a perceived or potential problem in that area. This may arise because of a problem the practice has actually experienced, e.g. several recent admissions of patients to hospital with hypoglycaemic attacks. This form of audit may be considered a 'critical incident method' (Berlin et al 1992). Following discussion with colleagues, it is decided to audit whether all doctors and community nurses attending patients in their own home have the equipment to deal with suspected hypoglycaemia.

Alternatively, another incentive to the audit process might be attendance at a course or the publication of a pertinent article.

Advice from national bodies such as the BDA, the RCN or the RCGP often suggests important topics which may be considered for audit. The Clinical Standards Advisory Group (1994) includes many suggestions for diabetic audit.

Likewise there are international targets established for standards of diabetic care. Any one of these standards may be selected to audit. The St Vincent Declaration establishes European goals for diabetic care and some of these are given in Box 8.4 (p. 180). It should be remembered however that the St. Vincent Declaration refers to very large population sizes so the outcomes it suggests may be impossible to assess at the general practice level.

The topics chosen for audit should be important enough to merit spending time and effort upon. Improvement should be considered achievable within a reasonable time frame.

All of this implies discussion with primary care team colleagues who will be affected by the result of the audit. It may be that only one community nurse and one doctor actually conduct the bulk of the work, but all clinical and administrative staff should be involved in the design of the audit process at an early stage. This is not for sentimental reasons. Only by involving the primary care team at an early stage can sufficient enthusiasm be generated to ensure change occurs.

WHICH CRITERIA SHOULD WE USE TO INVESTIGATE A TOPIC?

Even though staff choose to investigate a topic because of prompting from elsewhere, the criteria are likely to be generated internally. It is best to KISS (Keep It Short and Simple).

Choose one or two to begin with!

Most of the markers of good quality care are found to correlate highly within general practices (Farmer & Coulter 1990). If the practice is systematically checking visual acuity annually then it is probably getting the patients to take their shoes and socks off for a good foot examination.

Look for problems

If staff suspect that blood pressure recording is satisfactory, they should choose to look at another area, perhaps auditing the recording of smoking habits or whether educational efforts with diabetic smokers have been successful.

Case Study 11.2

The three topic areas for audit at the local Health Centre are registration, recall and regular eye checks. One of the doctors, a practice nurse and a district nurse agree to obtain relevant literature on the above topics. The team and one of the receptionists agree to meet to develop proposals for consideration by the whole practice team at the next practice meeting.

The practice agrees to establish criteria regarding structure, process and outcome.

Structure criteria for registration
- The practice has an active computerised diabetic register.
- The receptionist is familiar with the computer programme.
- There is table-top space for computer usage.
- Time is allocated for data entry.

Process criteria for registration
- The receptionist identifies all diabetic patients.
- The receptionist enters patient details onto the computer.
- The receptionist updates the computers on patient status.
- Adequate arrangements are made for backup of files.

Outcome criteria for registration
- Patients are identified as having diabetes.
- Patients' case notes are suitably marked to indicate that they have diabetes.
- Patient statistics are freely available for audit.

Further structure, process and outcome criteria are developed for the recall of patients and regular eye checks.

Staff then decide to audit the outcome criteria that 'Patients are identified as having diabetes'.

HOW DO WE SET STANDARDS THAT ARE RELEVANT IN OUR DAY-TO-DAY WORK?

Negotiate!

Decisions which affect everyone should involve everyone. Therefore decisions should be made at a regular practice meeting. If there are no regular meetings, then there is a problem. Success in audit is all about communication. If an audit of diabetic care is to be successful, staff must go to a meeting prepared to negotiate and discuss the topic, armed with facts and figures to support their case. They must encourage discussion to determine a mutually agreeable standard of care, resisting the temptation to say that every standard should be 100% right away. This would virtually guarantee that the goal will not be achieved. Realistic standards must be set which are fairly easy to achieve and which will maintain the motivation of the team.

In considering the criteria, there are few published standards for comparison. Therefore there are two options. The first option is to set the standard as part of a practice consensus. The second option is to collect the data and then decide the standard which staff would like to achieve on the next turn of the audit spiral. This latter option simplifies the decision about how much improvement is sought for the next time. For example if, as is likely, less than 50% of patients have had fundoscopy recorded either in hospital or in practice this year, then a goal might be suggested of 60% by next year and 100% in three years' time.

HOW CAN WE COMPARE OUR PERFORMANCE WITH THE SET STANDARDS?

We do this first by observing practice. This depends upon the area of care which staff wish to study and the criteria chosen. For some subjects one or two cases examined in detail may be enough: for example an audit into the prevention of hypoglycaemia. Staff could interview and review the casenotes of two patients recently admitted to hospital from the practice with hypoglycaemia to determine if these episodes could have been prevented. In other examples, adequate numbers of patients may be sampled from computer-generated lists. If nurses cannot coax the computer to produce these, they may have more success with the receptionists or the practice manager! Studies of insulin or oral hypoglycaemic prescribing can be done by using routinely generated data in the practice or from the local prescribing adviser. Box 11.2 gives a list of methods of data collecting which are readily available for audit.

Case Study 11.3

The nurses, the receptionist and the doctor sit down one afternoon, each with 10 case notes chosen at random from the computerised list of diabetic patients. They use an agreed method for extracting information on annual eye checks. They record the number of patients who have had an eye check and whether this has been at general practice, diabetic clinic, ophthalmology clinic or local optician. One of the nurses prepares a few simple pie charts, histograms or tables for distribution at the practice meeting.

Box 11.2 Methods of data collection	
Patients	Interview
	Questionnaire
Receptionists	Appointment book
	Access to lab reports/hospital
	Letters
Nurses	Access to nursing data
Casenotes	Review of specific diagnoses or drugs
Computer	Generates lists
	Some detailed analysis possible
Doctor	Carbon copies of prescriptions
Sources	Prescribing advisers
outside practice	Audit resource centres
	Primary care departments of Health Boards
	in FHSAs

The data collected should be believable. This means agreeing in advance with the practice what quality of data will persuade the other members of the primary care team to change. Advice is often available from audit facilitators but the following should be considered:

- Is the data collection method reliable?
- Is the data a complete or a representative sample?
- If sampling is used is it unbiased?

HOW DO THE FINDINGS FROM DATA COLLECTION COMPARE WITH THE SET STANDARDS?

Case Study 11.4

The first priority for the Health Centre is to improve its registration process (Kinmonth 1993). It is immediately obvious that they have fewer patients identified than would be expected from the known incidence of diabetes in their population. They have indentified 63 patients with diabetes. However, the known prevalence of diabetes in their population is 1.4% and hence they would have expected around 100 patients. The receptionist points out that some patients who come for urine testing strips are not on the list. Also patients with NIDDM controlled by diet were missed in this first search. In other words, not all patients with diabetes are on the register.

When reviewing the case notes, less than half had any record of eye checks during the previous 12 months. The records were incomplete for patients receiving solely GP care and also for patients attending the local hospital diabetic clinic. Was this poor recording, lack of communication, poor recall procedures or were patient default systems not being pursued?

The methods of analysis in audit need not be as complex as for research purposes. However the outcome of the audit and its implications should be clear for all to understand. This should be easily attained if simple criteria and definite standards are selected at the beginning of the audit. Box 11.3 shows the principal methods of

Box 11.3 Data interpretation	
• Quantitative	Numerical comparison Tables Histograms
• Qualitative	Sense of interviews Patient quotes Anecdotes

analysis. The quantitative approach gives numbers which can be compared and used to convince people of the need for improvement. Qualitative approaches give a depth of understanding. They also give explanations of why there are problems and often suggest ways of improvement.

HOW DOES DEMONSTRATING DEFICIENCIES HELP TO PRODUCE IMPROVEMENTS?

Case Study 11.5

The result were fed back to the full Practice meeting and an updated register and recall system was introduced. This was coordinated by the practice nurse who also involved all the doctors, the other community nurses, receptionists and local opticians to meet their set standards. A system was devised for reminding the community nurse that an annual eye check was due and the case notes were annotated to identify the patient as having diabetes. To determine the problem with those patients attending the hospital diabetic clinic, guidelines and protocols relating to communications were established.

Implementing change is the most difficult part of the project. However, the final hurdle may not be so bad if everyone has been involved in the process. Areas where improvements may be possible are often suggested by the process of investigation. If staff have chosen a good topic and studied it well enough to convince the rest of the practice that change is needed, they will be able to help identify ways of improvement.

> **Box 11.4**   Methods of improvement
>
> - Knowledge
> - Skills
> - Attitudes
> - Organisation

There are four areas which should be considered when attempting to generate improvements (Box 11.4). These are :

- **Knowledge**
  a) Which oral hypoglycaemic agents should be used in which circumstances?
  b) Does each doctor and community nurse have ready access to glucagon in surgery and on home visits?

- **Skills**
  a) Fundoscopy
  b) Instructing patients on urinalysis

- **Attitudes**
  a) Motivation in smoking cessation
  b) Importance of good glycaemic control

- **Organisation**
  a) Organised personal care
  b) Equipment.

IS AUDIT WORTHWHILE?

Yes. Practices who have published the results of audit have shown marked and sometimes dramatic improvements in care. These have been easier to demonstrate for measures of structure and process (Table 11.1, p. 234). However, there seems to be a clear link between such measures and outcome, and it is hoped that future editions of this book will contain shining examples of better outcomes for patients whose community nurses were convinced of the need to improve care through audit.

SUMMARY

Guidelines are the broad framework from which local protocols are developed. These protocols can be the record from which criteria are derived. The level of performance of the criteria is the set standard. Having agreed on the set standard, this can be audited to determine how effective patient care is and what improvements are necessary.

Through setting standards, observing practice, evaluating the information and thereafter implementing change, the ascending spiral of the audit cycle continues.

The primary health care team through good communication can make this happen. Community nurses are in a prime position to facilitate the audit cycle and, as a result, improve the level of care they provide to patients with diabetes.

Now for all those patients with asthma, epilepsy, rheumatism ...

REFERENCES

Berlin A, Spencer J A, Bhopal R S, van Zwannenberg T D 1992 Audit of deaths in general practice: pilot study of the critical incident technique. Quality Health Care 1:231–235
Clinical Standards Advisory Group 1994 Standards of clinical care for people with diabetes. HMSO, London
Clinical Resource and Audit Group (CRAG) 1993 Clinical guidelines. Scottish Office, Edinburgh
Farmer A, Coulter A 1990 Organisation of care for diabetic patients in general practice: influence on hospital admissions. British Journal of General Practice 40: 331:56–58
Field M J, Lohr K N 1990 Clinical practice guidelines: direction of a new programme. National Academy Press, Washington DC
Kendall H, Kitson A 1986 Setting standards. Nursing Times 82:35:29–31
Kemple T J, Hayter S R 1991 Audit of diabetes in general practice. British Medical Journal 302:451–453
Kinmonth A L (editorial) 1993 Diabetic care in general practice. British Medical Journal 306:599–600
Stearn R, Sullivan F M 1993 Should practice nurses be involved in diabetic care? British Journal of Nursing 2:952–957
Sullivan F M, Stearn R 1992 A community based audit of diabetes care in Lanarkshire. CRAG Occasional Paper 9. Scottish Office, Edinburgh
Working for Patients, Command Paper 555 1989 HMSO, London

The organisation of diabetic care

Derek Gordon   Joan McDowell

INTRODUCTION

The anxious man sitting in the surgery may have developed diabetes. With the information provided elsewhere in this book you should be able to confirm the diagnosis, plan his treatment and set out to prevent the complications of his disease with confidence. But who will be responsible for organising his care now and in the future? This may at first sight seem a simple question to answer. However, the organisation of diabetic care in the UK is complex and multilayered.

THE KEY PLAYERS

Standing centre stage will be the patient and his GP who assumes responsibility for this man's care. His management is initiated in the practice, his continuing care may be at the diabetic 'mini-clinic' and any referrals to other health care professionals are instigated by his GP. In other words, the GP has continuing responsibility for the patient's care from his first scream to his last croak!

Many patients prefer to be seen in the familiar surroundings of their own general practice. In recent years there has been a continuing trend for patients to be transferred from hospital-based clinics to mini-clinics in the primary care setting. The mini-clinic may be relatively cheap to run, and GPs now receive a financial incentive to set up chronic disease management clinics.

The success of such mini-clinics depends upon the enthusiasm, education and expertise of the clinical staff involved. Where infra-structure, training and audit are lacking, the clinical outcome of GP-based mini-clinics compares unfavourably with hospital-based clinics (Day et al 1987, Singh et al 1984). The government has recognised this fact and has stipulated that chronic disease management clinics should have a patient register and that outcome is audited. However, the government has not indicated how such a system should be policed and monitored.

The mini-clinic may be appropriate for some patients to attend solely. However, the GP may decide to share the care of the patients with the local hospital clinic. In order for such a system to operate effectively, close cooperation and liaison between the general practice and hospital are required. Some hospital clinics offer packages of services which they can provide to the local general practices, thus meeting the individual needs of each practice. Shared care requires time and effort to organise and good communication is essential be-tween GP and hospital consultant.

In this trio, it is important that the best care possible is offered to the patient and that he is not lost among the many fields of responsibility.

Let's change the scenario. The GP may decide that the diabetic care of the patient is the prerogative of the hospital consultant. The patient is referred to the hospital diabetic clinic and his future care thereafter managed by the hospital. The primary health care team receive reports on the patient's progress which alert them to changes in the patient's condition should concurrent medical interventions be required.

THE HEALTH CARE SUPPORT TEAM

If the patient and GP are singing in harmony then who is supporting them? For the GP mini-clinic to function adequately a full complement of health care-professionals is needed as support. The most important amongst these is probably the community nurse. Stearn & Sullivan (1993) have demonstrated that when practice nurses were involved in diabetic care the performance of the practice was significantly improved. There is a growing need for training of these nurses in diabetic care so that standards within practice can be further improved. Diabetes education for nurses throughout the UK is unfortunately very variable.

Further back-up to the diabetic service can be provided by the community dietitian and chiropodist. In addition the community pharmacist and social worker may be required for additional support.

WIDER SUPPORT SERVICES

The local team requires some support, which is available from the hospital diabetic service.

The traditional out-patient clinic is often busy and impersonal. Its long waiting times, short consultation times and frequent changes in junior staff have made it unpopular with patients. Education for patients has been piecemeal, often hurried and lacking in resources to facilitate it. In recent years the hospital diabetic service has changed considerably with the development of the diabetic centre.

The diabetic centre is often an allocated area specifically designed for diabetic consultation and education (Knight 1991). This provides the facilities and space which allow patients to receive professional education from other members of the diabetic team. The centre is more accessible to patients by offering, for example, an answerphone service, drop-in clinics, and daily chiropody and foot clinics. It often includes an area where patients can meet in groups for education sessions, demonstration purposes or self-help. The centre is also a rich educational resource for other health care team members.

The hospital diabetic service would include the diabetic nurse specialist, the dietitian, the chiropodist and the secretary to the centre. Behind these individuals a long list of health care professionals would make up the other areas of support, as illustrated in Figure 12.1.

For a team to function in harmony, a leader is necessary. Unfortunately there is some debate as to who this should be. The hospital consultant, by nature, assumes it is his/her responsibility to lead the team and organise the hospital diabetic service. The consultant is responsible for training the junior doctors and supervising other

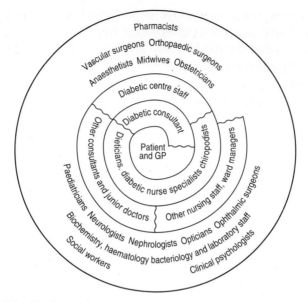

Fig. 12.1   The hospital diabetic service. The diabetic support network.

members of staff. Protocols for running the service and achieving standards of care should be produced. However, in this current climate of Trust hospitals, the general management team may well be the people who are calling the tune!

DIABETIC SUPPORT NATIONALLY

The work of the community and hospital diabetic teams is influenced by local, national and international bodies. These include the British Diabetic Association, the UK Government, the Clinical Standards Advisory Group and Local Advisory Groups, as well as international influences.

The British Diabetic Association

This consists of both amateur and professional contributors.

The British Diabetic Association was the first organisation in this country to involve both professional and lay people in the support of a particular patient group. The BDA has, since its inception, exerted powerful influence over all that encompasses diabetic care. Through its many sections and committees the BDA acts on behalf of patients, raises funds for research, promotes research and education and advises both the government and the medical profession on the allocation of resources to diabetic care and the organisation of that care.

The BDA is an independent registered charity and its income is obtained entirely from subscriptions obtained from its membership of 130 000 people and from voluntary donations. There are over 140 patient groups and branches throughout the UK which meet on a regular basis. These branches act as self-help groups and their members organise educational meetings as well as social events which can raise money for the Association.

The BDA has a commitment to education and training of not only the professionals and patients with diabetes but also the lay public. It produces a number of journals and magazines as well as a host of pamphlets and other educational material which are available to all interested parties.

The association's Medical and Scientific Section promotes research and arranges conferences which allow dissemination of the latest research information. Its membership is mainly medical and scientific staff. The Educational and Professional Care Section (EPCS) is responsible for promoting interest in these aspects of diabetic management. This section also holds a national conference. Membership of the EPCS is open to all health care professionals who choose to subscribe. It therefore provides a wide forum for debate and discussion on the care of patients with diabetes.

The BDA seeks to influence government and in particular the National Health Service. This involves the lobbying of policy makers, and contact with administrators and health care staff with the aim of educating, demonstrating needs and setting standards.

The government

The government has influenced diabetic care and provision by several different routes. Following the introduction of the new GP contracts in April 1990, 'new patient' registration medical examination became compulsory and this has introduced a screening programme for diabetes in the community. The GP contract also stipulates health checks every 3 years and the annual examination of all patients aged 75 years and older. While one might dispute the value of such routine checks, they have increased awareness of diabetes in the community and there is little doubt that many patients with un-recognised diabetes are identified by these routine examinations.

The government has greatly altered the organisation and structure of the NHS in recent years by introducing a purchaser-provider market for health care. Fund-holding general practices and local health authorities now contract for services from their local hospitals. They are therefore able to influence the type and scope of the services which can be provided by the hospital clinic or diabetic centre. Trust status for hospitals has provided a certain degree of uncertainty regarding the future funding of diabetic centres and the services that they provide. More than ever, it is important that management are aware of the need for both community and hospital care for patients with diabetes.

The government has identified the need for clinical guidelines and protocols in order to influence the practice of the medical, nursing and other health-related professions. In 1992 the Scottish Office published a working document which defined the terminology and set the agenda (Clinical Resource and Audit Group (CRAG) 1992). The development and implementation of guidelines has so far been slow. They are time-consuming and expensive to develop. A consensus within the profession may be difficult to obtain and unless guidelines are generally considered to be of value they will not be adhered to. Some fear that 'medicine by rote' will reduce the esteem of the profession and the clinical freedom of the doctor. A greater fear is that of litigation. Medical negligence arises when practitioners fall below the standards of care expected of their competent colleagues; if guidelines purport to embody these standards then justifying deviations from them would be difficult.

Clinical guidelines allow for standards to be set and for audit of those standards to be undertaken. The government can influence the implementation of guidelines and standards. For example, payment for chronic disease management clinics in general practice will only be provided in future if the practice can demonstrate that audit is proceeding. Similarly, it is likely that the purchasers of hospital diabetic care will increasingly demand evidence of ongoing audit and will include such stipulations in future contracts.

The Clinical Standards Advisory Group (CSAG)

The Clinical Standards Advisory Group was established in 1991 to advise the UK health ministers. 3 years later this group published its recommendations for standards of diabetic care in this country (Clinical Standards Advisory Group 1994). One of the most important recommendations of this group was the establishment of Local Diabetes Service Advisory Groups. These groups will be discussed in more detail below.

The CSAG produced 11 recommendations. Several of these relate to the contracting for and purchasing of adequate diabetic services. It emphasises that patients with diabetes should be involved in the development of the diabetic services.

CSAG also recognised the need for comprehensive diabetic registers to be established and maintained. Such registers would allow for monitoring of care quality and for assessing the health care needs of the local diabetic population. These registers would contain much clinical information on the health of diabetic patients and could be used for auditing standards. In order that all health care professionals can audit the same information, the need for a standard diabetic database has been recognised and the BDA in particular has been active in compiling such a database (Piwernetz et al 1993).

The CSAG report emphasised the need for cooperation between primary care sectors and hospitals for achieving optimum care for diabetics. The report also recognises the need for continuing education of all health care professionals associated with diabetic care and indeed the government has recognised the requirement to fund this education.

The report identifies the need for complications screening and for the organisation of health resources to reduce the risk of complications. In addition, prompt treatment facilities are required for such complications when they develop. In particular, screening for eye complications is highlighted.

Local Diabetes Service Advisory Groups (LDSAGs)

The establishment of LDSAGs was recommended in the CSAG-Diabetes report discussed above (CSAG 1994). Following the latest reorganisation of the NHS, responsibility for the allocation of health resources has been delegated to the Local Health Authorities or Health Boards. The LDSAGs are therefore of prime importance in ensuring that adequate resources are provided locally for the care of diabetic patients.

The membership of the LDSAGs is flexible but should contain a core group comprising members of the specialist diabetes team, local people with diabetes, members of the local Health Authority or Board, local fundholding GPs and local representatives of the BDA. In addition other interested members can be added to the Group as indicated by local circumstances (Box 12.1).

These groups will be responsible for planning the diabetic care of the local population and for establishing guidelines which govern that care. The presence of health authority and patient representatives on these bodies will ensure that their influence will also be exerted upon the type of diabetic care provided. They should take account of national and BDA guidelines as well as recommendations from other groups, such as the St Vincent Declaration (see below). They may also be responsible for education and training in diabetes locally and for audit and research.

The LDSAG should therefore advise on commissioning and contracting for diabetic services. It should also ensure that the diabetic

---

Box 12.1   Members of the Local Diabetes Service Advisory Groups

Core group
• The service providers with their managers:
  the hospital diabetes team—consultant, diabetic nurse specialist, dietitian, chiropodist
  the primary health care team—GP, community nurse specialist, community dietitian, chiropodist

• Local people with diabetes and their carers

• The service purchasers:
  representatives from the local health authority or board, fundholding GPs

• Local representatives of the BDA

Occasional members
Representatives of:
• Other clinical specialties
• Voluntary organisations
• Community health councils
• Ethnic minority groups
• Technical and scientific experts

services which are provided locally meet the needs and satisfy not only the health care professionals but also the patients.

INTERNATIONAL INFLUENCES ON DIABETIC CARE—THE ST VINCENT DECLARATION

Diabetic care in the UK is also affected by international decisions of which, in recent years, the St Vincent Declaration has been the most influential.

As described in earlier chapters, leading experts in diabetes met in St Vincent, Italy during 1989 in order to establish targets for the care of diabetic patients throughout Europe. The impetus for this meeting and the subsequent Declaration was the recognition that many health care systems were unaware of the consequences of diabetes on the health of the population. There was often an unawareness of modern developments in diabetes, the central role of the patient in the management of his or her own condition and the resultant need for patient education. The consequence of this ignorance has been a failure to achieve optimal levels of care. In addition it was widely recognised within the profession that the outcome of this care was rarely measured or assessed.

The St Vincent Declaration (WHO, International Diabetes Federation, 1989) is a document which sets standards for diabetic care and the time intervals for achieving them. A list of the most important health care targets is shown in Box 12.2. The Declaration also recognised the need to establish monitoring and control systems in order to record and subsequently audit clinical outcomes.

The UK Government has accepted the targets of the St Vincent Declaration and with the BDA has established the Joint Department of Health/BDA St Vincent Task Force. The purpose of the Task Force Group has been to recommend ways in which health resources can be organised in order to meet the targets of the Declaration. The first report of the Task Force identified those recommendations from the Declaration which should receive the highest priority (Box 12.3).

The Task Force has subsequently established a series of subgroups which include as members experts in a wide range of medical specialties associated with the care of diabetes and its complications. The remit of the subgroups is to provide detailed guidelines for

---

Box 12.2 Targets of the St Vincent Declaration

General goals
- Sustained improvement in health experience approaching normal.
- Prevention and cure of diabetes and its complications through intensive research.

Five year targets
- Introduce and evaluate comprehensive programmes for detection and control of diabetes and its complications.
- Raise awareness among the population and health care professionals of diabetes and its complications.
- Organise training and teaching in diabetes management.
- Ensure that children with diabetes receive care from professionals trained both in diabetes and paediatrics and that families receive adequate support.
- Reinforce existing centres and create new centres of excellence in diabetes.
- Promote independence and the fullest possible integration into society for all people with diabetes.
- Reduce blindness due to diabetes by one third or more.
- Reduce end-stage diabetic renal failure by at least one third.
- Reduce by one half the rate of limb amputations for diabetic gangrene.
- Cut morbidity and mortality from coronary heart disease by rigorous programmes of risk factor reduction.
- Achieve diabetic pregnancy outcome similar to that of the nondiabetic.
- Establish monitoring and control systems using state-of-the-art information technology.
- Promote international programmes for diabetes research.

Box 12.3 St Vincent Task Force priorities

- monitoring and control systems for diabetes
- planning, provision and audit of services
- special needs for children and adolescents
- patient-centred care
- education and training
- preventing blindness
- preventing renal complications
- preventing foot complications
- preventing coronary heart disease
- preventing pregnancy complications
- research and development

Box 12.4   The St Vincent Task Force subgroups

- cardiovascular disease
- children and young people
- clinical care
- diabetic foot and amputation
- education and training
- information and epidemiology

- patients and carers
- pregnancy and neonatal care
- renal disease
- research and development
- visual impairment

---

achieving the targets of the St Vincent Declaration. A list of the subgroups set up in England and Wales is shown in Box 12.4. Similar subgroups have been established in Scotland. Guidelines for the implementation of the St Vincent Declaration have been produced (Krans et al 1995), and further guidelines will follow.

It has been recognised by the Task Force that patients themselves should have a say in the provision of the type of service provided for them. Education of both patients and those responsible for their care has also been recognised as of primary importance. There is a recognition of the special needs of younger and older people with diabetes and those from different ethnic backgrounds.

THE CONCERTED EFFORT

The provision of diabetic care in the UK is complex and in constant flux. The GP has taken on more responsibility in recent years for the continuing care and surveillance of diabetic patients within the primary care setting. Behind the GP stands a vast array of medical and paramedical support both within the community and also the hospital service. In order to achieve optimal diabetic care it is necessary for cooperation between GPs, community and hospital services who should work together to provide 'shared care'.

Powerful influences upon the service are exerted from Government bodies, the BDA and international bodies. Great emphasis is placed at present on the requirement to set standards of care and to monitor and measure clinical outcomes so that all patients throughout the UK can expect the best possible care of their diabetes and its complications. The St Vincent Task Force has emphasised the central role of the patient, who should take increasing responsibility for his/her own

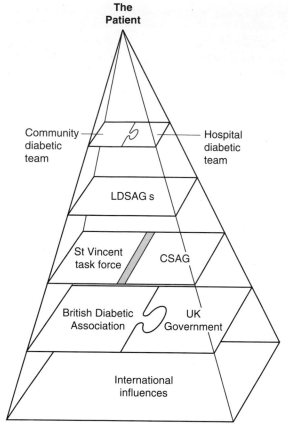

Fig. 12.2 The organisation of diabetic care.

diabetic care. In this complex system, which has developed for organising diabetic care it is important not to lose sight of the key player, the patient.

REFERENCES

Clinical Standards Advisory Group Subcommittee on Diabetes 1994 Standards of clinical care for people with diabetes. Dept of Health/HMSO, London

Clinical Resource and Audit Group (CRAG) 1992 Moving to audit. What every doctor needs to know about medical audit. University of Dundee/Clinical Resource and Audit Group

Day J L, Humphreys H, Alban-Davies H 1987 Problems of comprehensive shared diabetes care. British Medical Journal 294:1590–1592

Knight A H 1991 Organisation of diabetes care in the hospital. In: Pickup J C, Williams G (eds) Textbook of diabetes. Blackwell Scientific, Oxford

Krans H M J, Porta M, Keen H, Staehr Johansen K 1995 Diabetes care and research in Europe: the St Vincent Declaration action programme. Implementation document. World Health Organization, Rome

Piwernetz K, Home P D, Snorgaard O, Antsiferov M, Staehr Johansen K, Krans M 1993 Monitoring the targets of the St Vincent Declaration and the implementation of quality management in diabetes care: the DiabCare Initiative. Diabetic Medicine 10:371–390

Singh B M, Holland M R, Thorn P A 1984 Metabolic control of diabetes in general practice clinics: comparison with a hospital clinic. British Medical Journal 289:726–728

Stearn R, Sullivan F M 1993 Should practice nurses be involved in diabetic care? British Journal of Nursing 2:952–957

World Health Organization (Europe) and International Diabetes Federation (Europe) 1980 Diabetes mellitus in Europe: a problem at all ages in all countries—a model for prevention and self care. WHO, St Vincent

Index

Page numbers in bold type refer to illustrations, boxes and tables.